UNDERSTANDING
HOMOEOPATHY

UNDERSTANDING HOMOEOPATHY

Dr. Trevor Smith

M.A., M.B.Chir., D.P.M., M.F.Hom.

INSIGHT

Insight Editions
WORTHING, Sussex
1987

First published 1983

Revised 1987

© Trevor Smith 1987

British Library Cataloguing in Publication Data

Smith, Trevor, *1934–*
   Understanding homoeopathy.—2nd ed.
   1. Homoeopathy
   I. Title
   615.5′32   RX71

ISBN 0-946670-12-9

WARNING
The contents of this volume are for general interest only and
individual persons should always consult their medical
adviser about a particular problem or before stopping or
changing an existing treatment.

Printed and bound in Great Britain by
Biddles, Guildford, Surrey

Contents

		Page
	Introduction	ix
1	What is homoeopathy – some initial definitions and explanations	1
2	Origins	14
3	The homoeopathic conception of illness and disease	21
4	The basic causation of illness	36
5	The indications for homoeopathy	59
6	The action and functions of homoeopathy	75
7	Dilution and disease	89
8	The advantages of the homoeopathic approach	94
9	Some limitations	103
10	More indications for homoeopathy	106

v

11	Preparation of the remedies	115
12	Making a start	119
13	Homoeopathy and the home	127
14	First aid	133
15	The twenty basic remedies and their usage	150
16	Some useful addresses and places of contact	163
	Recommended reading	166
	Index	167

In Homoeopathy, the aim is clarity of diagnosis and knowledge of the total person as an aid to understanding all the relevant factors which cause or contribute to the illness.

Introduction

The chapters which follow are written for the general reader as well as the interested patient and family who want to learn more about the homoeopathic approach to illness, prevention and cure.

The book aims to inform as well as to stimulate interest, so that the reader can try out for himself some of the remedies discussed for the simple everyday problems which occur daily in every family and which do not require conventional medical help or emergency treatment.

Homoeopathy often has the edge over the conventional approach for the common conditions which only require simple relief of pain and discomfort. More and more people are resisting the overwhelming approach of conventional drugs for ordinary problems because they know how depleting and exhausted they can feel as a result.

Because homoeopathy only gives a natural and specific biological stimulus back to health, the patient does not have to cope with side-effects, nor do the remedies leave the patient feeling jaded and confused, worse than the condition which required help in the first place.

Homoeopathy is on the side of the patient because it is safe and without risk as long as the method is used sensibly and appropriately.

I recommend that the book be read at least once in its totality and then the reader can return to the more specialised chapters of personal interest.

Use the book as a practical reference guide, keeping it by the side of your homoeopathic medical box where it is handy and available when a remedy is needed.

Also use the margins of the book to make notes on any remedies tried, with their results and the date.

When properly stored, in a cool dry place away from perfumes, cosmetics, menthol and camphor, the remedies keep indefinitely without losing their efficiency. In this way they are always available for action and effect when needed. Make the book work for you as you gain experience and knowledge by working through the recommended remedies.

CHAPTER ONE

Some initial definitions and explanations

Homoeopathy is a prescribable treatment for a wide variety of illnesses using extracts of natural substances chosen and prepared for the patient in a way that is unique in medicine. The basic materials come from a wide variety of sources.

The majority are those of plant origin – for example *Calendula* (Marigold), *Convalaria maj.* (Lily of the Valley), *Bryonia* (Hop), *Hydrastis* (Golden Seal), *Digitalis* (Foxglove), *Lilium tig* (Tiger Lily), *Pulsatilla* (Anenome or Wind Flower), *Avena sat* (Common Oat).

Others are of insect origin. Some of the commonest include *Apis* (Bee), *Blatta* (Cockroach), *Formica rufa* (Ant), *Cantharis* (Spanish Fly), *Pulex Irritans* (Flea). Spider remedies include *Theridion* (Orange spider), *Mygale lasiodora* (Black Cuban spider), *Latrodectus mactans* (Black Widow spider), *Tarentula hispania* (Spanish spider), *Cedron aranea diadema* (Papal-Cross spider).

Snake remedies are made up from venom and include *Naja tripudians* (Cobra), *Cenchris Contortrix* (Copperhead snake), *Lachesis* (Bushmaster snake), *Crotalus horridus* (Rattlesnake), *Bothrops lanciolatus* (Yellow Viper).

Yet other remedies come from the sea including *Medusa* (Jellyfish), *Trachinus* (Stingfish), *Murex* (Purple fish), *Sepia* (Cuttlefish), *Corallium* (Red Coral), *Ambra grisea* (Whale), *Fucus vesiculosus* (Sea Kelp), *Leum jecoris aselli* (Cod-liver Oil).

In addition there are important remedies called nosodes, acting like vaccines, but without their risks and side-effects. These are prepared from diseased tissue or cellular material. For example *Pertussin* used in the treatment and prevention of whooping cough is made from the mucus of throat swabs of whooping cough sources. In addition *Diptherinum* (potentized Dipheria Virus) is useful in Diptheria-like conditions, or when there is an epidemic when it can be used prophylactically. Other nosodes include *Influenzinum* (Potentized Influenza virus), *Morbillinum* (Measles), *Varicellinum* (Potentized Chicken Pox virus), *Rubellinum* (German Measles), *Tuberculinum* (from Tubercular Morbid material), *Medorrhinum* (Gonorrhoeal virus). All can be of enormous value in the treatment and prevention of the conditions mentioned.

Other remedies have a particular action on various organs and their function. Mobility remedies include *Rhus tox* (Poison Ivy), *Bryonia* (Wild Hop), *Ruta graveolens* (Rue), *Rhododendron* (Snow-Rose), *Dulcamara* (Bitter Sweet).

Some respiratory remedies acting strongly on

2

lung function are *Lycopodium* (Club Moss), *Arsenicum album* (Arsenic Trioxide), *Natrum sulph* (Sulphate of Sodium), *Bryonia* (Wild Hop), *Phosphorus*.

Other excretory remedies acting on the kidney organs or kidney function are *Berberis vulgaris* (Barberry), *Cantharis* (Spanish Fly) and *Natrum muriaticum* (Chloride of Sodium).

Circulatory remedies act on the heart, circulation and fluid balance. These include *Pulsatilla* (Wind Flower), *Apis* (Bee), *Cactus grandiflorus* (Night-blooming Cireus), *Convallaria* (Lily of the Valley), *Spigelia* (Pinkroot), *Digitalis* (Foxglove), *Aurum metallicum* (Metallic Gold).

Homoeopathy finds its origin in classical Greek and its roots *homeos* and *pathos*, mean 'equal suffering'. This gives the clue to the action and approach of the method which is to treat 'suffering' or illness using remedies that in their natural, unprepared state can produce 'equal' or similar physical and psychological symptoms to those of the patient.

In general, homoeopathy uses substances which in their raw original state have the ability to violently irritate, inflame or stimulate a physiological reaction in various parts of body and organ functioning. The remedies act on areas where they have been applied locally, but also more widely too. This innate power of the Mother substance to stimulate the organism, is preserved and carried through into the remedies by the homoeopathic pharmacist's unique way of preparing the potencies by serial dilution and succession. In this way the original energy is still available but in a more

3

controlled way for the patient, to form an intrinsic part of the remedies' potential to treat and cure.

Deadly Nightshade for example, from which the remedy *Belladonna* is prepared, when taken in its crude form from the hedgerow, produces an intensely toxic reaction. There is collapse, burning pains, a flushed red face, dilated pupils and a bounding pulse. The temperature is raised and nausea or vomiting are frequently apparent. The least jolt or movement may aggravate all the symptoms. This poison-reaction closely resembles the clinical picture of severe scarlet-fever which also has a scalding skin rash, a raised temperature and burning pains – susceptible to jarring, noise or disturbance of any kind. Such clinical symptoms clearly resemble the toxic manifestations of *Belladonna* before it is extracted from Deadly Nightshade and it is this *similarity* which is used as the underlying principle when choosing a remedy to treat and cure a particular type of scarlet fever response.

Other remedies for severe Scarlet fever are *Aconitum napellus* (Monkshood) the skin is hot, dry and burning, but in contrast to *Belladonna* where the patient lies prostrated, the least movement aggravates. When *Aconitum* is indicated there is marked restlessness coupled with intense fear and anxiety. *Rhus tox* (Poison Ivy) is indicated for a milder illness with intense itching where the patient feels better for both warmth and movement. *Stramonium* (Thorn Apple) is indicated for more severe cases with high fever, the body covered with profuse sweating and delirium is a feature. The typical restless agitation is aggravated

4

by the sight of water or when the light is switched off. *Ammonium carb* (Carbonate of Ammonia) is for a more malignant form of the disease with fluid retention but only a mild burning or itching rash. Drowsiness or a heavy feeling is marked, the throat severely painful. *Muriaticum acidum* (Muriatic Acid) is indicated for weakness and collapse, the pulse rapid and weak and when haemorrages occur. *Lachesis* (Bushmaster Snake) is prescribed for a purplish or blueish rash. All the symptoms are worse after sleep and accompanied by an intolerance of the least form of pressure from sheets or clothing. *Ailanthus glandulosa* (Chinese Sumach) has a dark purple rash, the throat swollen and red. Prostration, drowsiness, weakness and diarrhoea are also present when this remedy is needed.

Research studies called 'provings', toxicity recordings and clinical experience are all used to form an overall symptom-profile for each remedy which provides an accurate prediction of the one most likely to be effective at any given time. Such proving profiles are traditionally built-up by listing the overall portrait of symptoms developed by a group of healthy volunteers who have been taking a particular 'un-named' remedy for several weeks. Usually one member of the proving group is especially sensitive to the chosen potency, adding to the general reaction patterns which evolve and giving a more specific description to the remedy tested. He or she may develop an odd, rare or peculiar response to the proving substance – for example the sensation that the intestines are made of glass *Thuja* (Tree of Life). In a proving experiment carried out by the author using *Kali carb* (Carbonate of Potassium) one person out of twelve was especially sensitive and developed key diagnostic symptoms of swelling of the upper eyelids during the experiment. Other members of the trial developed a more overall profile of the remedy. Together these created the total picture of the remedy as is recorded in the repertory and used when evaluating which remedy is best suited for a particular patient.

There is still controversy among homoeopaths and critics of the method, as to the value and even relevance of these original provings carried out by Hahnemann and his colleagues. Often quite small groups of volunteers were used in the early days, using colleagues, family or friends in the first trials. It has been suggested that these were unscientific or are invalid because of the small numbers and the absence of more modern sophisticated techniques as double-blind or cross-over methods, not developed at that time. But for the practicing homoeopath what matters is not whether the original experiments were consistent or even scientific, but whether they have clinical application and relevance to the patient, reliability as a working method and are safe.

In practice, despite the historical nature of the early provings, some of which have not been repeated, the remedies have been consistently and widely used by homoeopaths in every country with positive results. Clinical experience over the years gives security to both patient and doctor alike, when a curative reaction is being sought, whatever the scientific validity of the method or its adherance to statistics, current theory and research practice.

Matching a contemporary symptom or disease with the patterns of a historical proving may at first sight seem illogical, but however enigmatic the early proving experiments, the results have consistently stood the test of time over the years. For most physicians, this is a satisfactory indication and confirmation of which remedy to prescribe.

For these reasons, the classical repertory is still the best reference point for the homoeopath, at least until a new or better list of indications is evolved. In general any re-proving experiments have largely confirmed the original findings of the early provers.

However Homoeopathy is not primarily concerned with an automatic-cure for a condition as scarlet-fever, but seeks to treat and support the variety of individual responses to their condition, varying enormously from one person to another. This concern for the individual and his unique patterns of response is characteristic of the whole homoeopathic approach. *Belladonna* may be perfectly appropriate for one member of the family with a severe and toxic scarlet fever illness, but in another, the reaction may be quite different. The rash may be mild – the predominant problem a chest condition with a dry irritating cough preventing sleep, so that *Bryonia* – the extract of the wild hop is more needed. In another child, the throat is the major problem but without either a toxic state, severe rash or involvement of the chest. Where the throat is purple so that the least swallowing becomes painful and agonising, then neither of these two remedies is appropriate and *Phytolacca* – the extract of the poke-root plant is indicated –

however much *Belladonna* is considered as the specific for scarlet-fever. In the final clinical analysis, it is always the individual symptom-pattern and the patient that decides the remedy, not a diagnostic label, clinical entity or 'scientific' theoretical treatment, leading to a theoretical, non-personal approach and practice of medicine.

Homoeopathy is more than just an effective treatment for the individual. It is an overall way of looking at the patient. Every aspect of the person is taken into account when assessing and considering the most appropriate remedy for a problem and one likely to help. However physical the complaint – perhaps a problem of eczema, hiatus hernia, 'blood pressure', varicose veins or haemorrhoids, the patient's psyche and psychological make-up is always considered in detail as part of understanding the totality of the illness and totality of make-up.

Homoeopathy's major concern is stimulation of the individual's overall response and a more balanced functioning of the internal organs, to build-up of vitality and reserves. This overall functioning of the patient is taken into account each time a remedy is prescribed, with attention to both physical and psychological areas of concern or pre-occupation by the individual.

But homoeopathy is more than just a simple treatment of illness. It is also an effective diagnostic approach to the individual as a unique entity in his own right, based on how the person is feeling at the time, in the consulting room *now*, and not in a remote past situation. Remedies are about curing present-day problems and are diagnosed by the symptoms and awareness of the patient as they are evolving, and changing.

Every patient is more than just a collection of symptoms and clinical signs. He is also a human being with feelings, sensitivity and vulnerability, having to cope daily with stress, decision-making and problem-solving often at complex levels. The reason or trigger to illness and why the body's defences have failed or become overwhelmed is always of concern to the practicing homoeopath and frequently the first remedy goes back to treat these depths and causes.

Homoeopathy offers a safe total treatment because it also compliments the individual, giving a gentle stimulus to vitality and wholeness. Homoeopathy looks at the present as well as at the past. It considers the reasons how and where a particular remedy can help modify or absorb the remnants of an earlier traumatic situation which still exists as an unresolved irritant – either physically or psychologically within the person.

Each remedy is assessed for the treatment of both outer external manifestations of dysfunction and for any underlying, more subtle pressures and distortions which contribute to it. The causes of many illnesses have their origins in the past, with symptoms no more than the tip of the iceberg. To be really effective, the homoeopathic remedy needs to treat the deepest causes as well as the clinically obvious. As in the The Time Machine of H. G. Wells, the higher potencies can fortunately transcend time and work backwards as well as in the present to clear and reverse undesirable past patterns and trends, damaged areas of disharmony which over the years have contributed to a jaded state of chronic ill health.

Only homoeopathy has this unique dual-action. The well-prescribed remedy sweeps backwards and horizontally in time back to the origins of a complaint, often through several generations, at the same time striking vertically to reach the emotional and physical layers of the prevailing symptoms.

However psychological, or obviously emotional a problem – anxiety-tension, depression, agitation state or insomnia difficulty, the patient's physical health should be given equal weight as the more obvious psychological aspects. This includes reserves and energy, physiological patterns and body rhythms, to give an overall picture with maximum of information in all areas.

In homoeopathy the aim is clarity of diagnosis and knowledge of the total person as an aid to understanding all the relevant factors which cause or contribute to the illness. The practitioner can then choose a remedy which closely matches the patient's overall psychological and physical profile.

Homoeopathy is also a philosophy of cure in the sense that it doesn't regard disease as an illness arriving and implanting itself in an unsuspecting organ or cellular area of the body. The whole disease-process is seen as part of an overall totality in the development and evolution of the individual, so that his or her vulnerability and susceptibility at that particular time has sense and meaning. Illness is usually far more than just a passive act of infiltration by a virus organism or simple invasion by a 'germ' – whatever form it takes. In most cases, the illness or disease is not an act of chance or a blow-of-fate which happened on one recognizable occasion, but relates to an overall state of both body and mind.

Often over a period of months or even years preceding an acute illness, there has been a whole chain of minor problems. These were not necessarily illnesses-in-themselves, but pointers that all was not right within, as abnormal susceptibility and weakness developed externally. The eventual illness is often the end-product of a succession of depleting events – both psychological as well as physical.

Homoeopathy puts a lot of emphasis on the mental attitudes of the individual, the underlying emotional health and satisfactions of the individual. Whatever the problem, it has always been considered of fundamental importance to help both the deeper aspects as well as the more apparent physical external symptoms and events. The remedies act very deeply in this psychological sphere and it is one of their major advantages, since when properly prescribed, homoeopathy helps both areas in depth.

Case report

A woman aged 55 came for a consultation. I had previously treated her, but had not seen her for the past six months. There had never been any previous history of skin troubles and in the past she had come with a joint or rheumatic problem (*Rhus tox*, *Medorrhinum*, *Pulsatilla*, *Dulcamara*, *Rhododendron*). This time there were none of her usual

11

symptoms and instead she complained of an odd, but severe irritating facial rash (*Sulphur*, *Urtica*, *Rhus tox*), which caused intolerable itching and discomfort. The symptoms were mainly over the left side of the face (*Belladonna*, *Apis*, *Lachesis*, *Pulsatilla*) and to a lesser extent over her whole body (*Sulphur*, *Psorinum*). The problem was present most of the day but definitely aggravated by heat and the warmth of the bed clothes (*Pulsatilla*, *Sulphur*, *Arg. nit.*).

There was not much to go on as far as diagnostic causes were concerned and she associated the rash with the use of a detergent and also a household-name natural bath-foam and soap which she had used frequently over the years. The condition became severe when she had worn a pair of woollen socks, washed in her usual detergent, but in her opinion, probably not sufficiently and thoroughly rinsed.

It seemed a great mystery. I then said that in all allergic cases, although a disease was not psychological in itself, nevertheless there was often an underlying psychological component which acted as a trigger to the more acute allergic reaction to surface. My patient thought for a moment and then after a meaningful pause said – 'well, during the period of the skin trouble, I very nearly lost my daughter-in-law and her baby from severe blood-pressure'. She had been in hospital at the time and there was certainly a great deal of worry and stress which she had not previously admitted to (*Aconitum*, *Natrum mur.*, *Lycopodium*, *Ignatia*).

Whether the emotion referred to was *the* causative factor is difficult to prove – it seems both possible and likely. It is interesting that she only gave the information about deeper psychological matters in response to my comments and the role of emotion in allergy. The case illustrates the close links between physical and deeper psychological happenings – not always admitted or recognizable to the patient.

As a matter of interest, the remedy emerging from the material given is likely to be either *Sulphur* or *Pulsatilla*, the former having stronger skin affiliations than the latter. In order to be quite certain as to which remedy is the 'right' one, you would need more information from the case history and details of the modalities.

CHAPTER TWO

Origins

Samuel Hahnemann, (1755–1843) physician and founder of homoeopathy was born in Meissen Southern Germany where both his father and grandfather had worked as artists to the local china industry. The family background may have contributed in some measure to his sensitive temperament and cultural interests as well as to Hahnemann's ability for attention to detail in his later research work. Always interested in the metaphysical and the arts, a close friend and admirer of Goëthe during later mature years, his temperament was well suited to accepting the indefinable, the mysterious and the incomplete. This was inevitable over prolonged periods while he was developing the homoeopathic approach and philosophy. Opposed to the crude often primitive approach to the patient which was prevalent at the time, Hahnemann disliked labelling a patient or naming a quick diagnosis or treatment. Throughout his life he was a vigorous opponent of indiscriminant suppressant physical treatments, especially blood-letting, purgation, the use of emetics and restraint.

This combination of linguistic gifts, medical background, sensitivity and patience, led him to develop ancient medical principles, known since Hipocrates, into a comprehensive science with a new and broad-ranging practical application for doctor and patient.

In his philosophical approach to treatment, he was closely allied in thought to the sixteenth century scholar Paracelsus, who doubtless had a considerable effect on the developing young Hahnemann.

Hippocrates, the Greek Physician and Father of modern scientific medicine, was born in Kos in 460BC. Gifted with vision and foresight, he emphasised the impossibility of understanding the functioning of the body without at the same time understanding the nature of the patient – as a whole person. Medicine and philosophy, the tangible and intangible, were combined in his new radical approach which stated that diseases have an understandable logic, a cause and period of aggravation or crisis which leads on to cure or a decline in the patient's condition. By seeing disease as a disturbance within the patient's constitution he anticipated modern concepts of illness where stress for example, is a major cause of dis-equilibrium. For Hippocrates, illness was caused by related or similar things – not something in isolation from the patient's totality and by using them in treatment, the patient could be cured. He recommended treating vomiting by using emetics, a febrile state by warm beverages or tepid bathing. These axioms of the greatest Greek Physician four centuries before

Christ, anticipated homoeopathy and the conclusions of Hahnemann in the 18th century – but there was a gap of nearly two thousand years before they were fully developed.

Paracelsus (1490–1541) the European physician, philosopher and alchemist also emphasised that what makes man ill can also cure – provided it is given in a small enough dose. He is reputed to have had outstanding results in the plague epidemic of 1534 by administering a 'pill' made of bread and minute pin-head amounts of the patient's excreta.

Hahnemann was medically qualified at the age of 24, working first as a linguist, translating and teaching. He travelled widely gaining medical experience and also studying as a botanist. But after nearly a decade of practice he became disenchanted with conventional medical approaches which he regarded as barbaric and devoted himself entirely to writing and translation work. One of his earliest papers is about the toxic effects of arsenic poisoning and this may have influenced his thinking when it was later developed as a major polycrest or multiple-acting remedy (*Arsenicum*).

During his period of withdrawal from formal medical practice, Hahnemann became deeply involved with translating The Materia Medica of the Scottish physician Cullen who by 1789 had completed a second edition. Hahnemann became dissatisfied with what Cullen had written about malaria and the way that quinine acted. He had a practical knowledge of the illness from clinical work in the Low Countries shortly after qualifying. This dissatisfaction led to a series of practical

16

experiments, and the insights which developed to the birth of homoeopathy.

Hahnemann decided to test the result of quinine (Cinchona bark) on himself using the tincture. Although perfectly healthy at the time, within hours he developed the symptoms of a malaria-like illness with intermittent fever, chilly extremities, prostration, drowsiness and flushed cheeks. These symptoms disappeared as soon as he ceased taking quinine. From such first experiments, Hahnemann developed the basic concept of using a natural substance in the treatment of illness which in its raw state can produce similar effects to those of the illness. He described these radical new concepts and the philosophy of their action in the Organon (1810). This was to be his most important book and is still a classic and source of reference, particularly the later sixth edition.

Similar principles can be seen in primitive tribes. Fear of the wrath of omnipotent gods was appeased by creating fearsome replicas, especially masks and totums of awesome figures in order to avoid their feared retributions. In primitive communities, action to avoid the threat of drought or flooding is sometimes taken by the local power or medicine man who 'creates' by ritualistic dance – catastrophes-in-miniature, to bring urgently needed rain, or conversely to subdue swollen rivers. The old principle of 'a hair of the dog', known for generations, is giving a little more of what has already been experienced and caused discomfort.

Until recently and certainly prior to the pharmaceutical 'revolution', homoeopathy was the normal approach to health and used by all doctors. Even today it is still quite common to meet patients who can clearly recall taking *Arnica* for bruising and *Rhus tox* for sprains as a child, the whole family treated homoeopathically.

Initially Hahnemann found that using the undiluted mother tinctures in treatment could sometimes provide toxic effects in his patients although the indications were correct and the remedies were being given homoeopathically.

Hahnemann experimented by diluting the tinctures to the point where they could be given more safely without losing their therapeutic potential. To his amazement, dilution did not diminish the power of the remedies but on the contrary increased their scope and depth of action. The greater the dilution the more powerful and effective the remedy. Succussion, or vigorous shaking of each dilution is essential to 'stamp' the therapeutic qualities upon the solution, also one of Hahnemann's fundamental and unique discoveries.

Nevertheless, Hahnemann was often consulted by patients where the remedies, even in their diluted dynamised form were without lasting effect. These were the problems of chronic illness and Hahnemann worked for many years on such difficulties, culminating in his volume 'Chronic Diseases' which set out his new theories of miasms. The miasm is the 'ghost' of the original illness. He grouped chronic illness into three main headings due to miasms, which he saw as containing certain characteristics of an original earlier illness occurring within a family, perhaps over several generations. Psora is the most widespread and important, linked to earlier scabies or 'the itch'. Sycosis was related to Gonorrhoeal disease in an earlier generation and Syphilis to a previous syphilitic infection affecting subsequent generations to some degree. This was the theory and not everyone accepted it, but it nevertheless provides a useful way of analysing current problems of chronic illness. The major remedies associated with the miasmic illness are for Psora – *Sulphur*, for Sycosis – *Thuja* and for Syphilis – *Mercurius*.

From the onset Hahnemann opposed his patients using any form of violent stimulant or dietary excess during their treatment. He condemned alcohol, tea or coffee and also the use of lead plasters and ointments, although popular at the time. He recommended strict standards of diet, hygiene and regular exercise, emphasising a positive attitude for physician and patient. He advised avoidance of stimulant spices or herbs, which have a marked physiological action, especially during an acute illness. These included pepper, curry and peppermint during homoeopathic treatment. He also advocated a salt-free diet if *Mercurius* was prescribed and a low intake of acid foods with *Belladonna*, *Aconite* and *Digitalis*.

As a young physician, Hahnemann worked in mental institutions with the problems of psychological illness. He wrote several articles recommending a more friendly humanitarian approach to build up greater confidence within the patient. He wanted remedies kept to a strict minimum and abandoned the usual practice of prescribing vast quantities of multiple drugs (or polyprescribing). He gave priority to the patient's individual constitution and needs, contacts with the family, moderation, regular exercise, diet and fresh air. In this way Hahnemann stressed the importance of looking at the patient as part of the family and his or her social constellation, anticipating the importance of 'family therapy'.

Hahnemann also examined ecological issues, especially pollution for which he gave specific recommendations that his patients avoid strong odours or fumes from stoves or fumigators. He thought it ill-advised for patients to have plants or flowers in the rooms but above all he emphasised the needs of each individual to have their personal 'space' or area around them – to create confidence and for unrestricted movement. These recommendations were combined with a healthy balanced diet, the specific homoeopathic remedy and were revolutionary at that time.

In his more general writings, Hahnemann opposed all pressure on the individual. Woman's lib. was not yet known – but he recommended that girls should be brought up to be themselves with a natural upbringing, criticising pressures or patterns of any sort which might impart an artificial or masculinising effect upon their vulnerable and developing personality.

For certain illnesses he also recommended an exclusion diet – eliminating for example, potatoes from the diet of asthmatics. Contemporary skin sensitivity tests support his hypothesis with many patients showing hypersensitivity to potato or the related nightshade plants – egg plant and tomato, because of the toxic responses they engender in certain sensitive patients.

CHAPTER THREE

The Homoeopathic conception of disease and illness

For centuries philosophers have seen man as a microcosm of the universe – not only a reflection but in relationship with it. By his habits and patterns, periods of energy-spurts and activity, the need for quiet, hibernation and withdrawal, man has natural rhythms and seasons of growth. These lead on to maturity and a harvesting of fruits – not only of physical labour but also of thought and well-being.

Man contains many polarities and contrasts within his make-up to give a balanced overall relationship between tonicity and relaxation, psychological and physical; instinct and impulse; logic and intuitiveness; thought and emotion; consciousness and unconsciousness; mature sensitivity and infantile demands of self-interest; need of others – for love, protection and closeness contrasting with impulses to control hurt, separate, domi-

21

nate and to impose upon.

To some degree all of these are present in everyone, within a fluid changing configuration of maturity and health. Each contributes something to the overall whole, the psychological totality, as well as to constitutional identity. In health, no one aspect dominates or overwhelms another, although one feature – for example, fear or apprehension, may temporarily intrude and take over at times of a particular stress or pressure, but not in a permanent way. These various aspects of the human constellation, form the parimeters, or characteristics of individuality, expressed as patterns of response, vitality, aims, drive and priorities which motivate towards success and failure, sickness or health.

These characteristics are constantly used by the homoeopath as the guiding modalities or modifying features, the constitutional patterns of variation of individuality reflecting the essence of the person and showing which particular remedy is most indicated at the time. Intensity, or a build-up of pressure, in a particular area of expression, and functioning is usually experienced as a particular need or symptom-pattern. For example a rheumatic pain may be better for warmth and exercise, indicating *Rhus tox*, or a stress situation with agitation and a craving for warmth and affection, suggests *Phosphorus*. When the symptoms however are worse for exercise or warmth, then *Bryonia* is most likely to be the remedy of choice. If the rheumatism is more a reflection of psychological insecurity and stiffness, then *Natrum mur.* may be the remedy indicated.

22

In health, man is centred, in a position of balance, a dynamic combination of tonicity and relaxation, not just simply one fixed in tension or passivity. There is a *gentle* awareness, without suppression, an unconscious knowing that the heart is beating without palpitation (*Spigelia*, *Digitalis*, *Convallaria*, *Aurum met*, *Naja trip*, *Spongia tosta*), the lungs functioning without breathlessness *Arsenicum*, *Natrum sulph*, *Phosphorus*, *Medorrhinum*), the limbs moving without stiffness (*Rhus tox*, *Causticum*, *Rhododendron*, *Dulcamara*).

The balanced body surface contains a sufficient quantity of moisture without drenching sweats (*Silicea*, *Calcarea*, *Thuja*, *Aconitum*, *Pulsatilla*) or unpleasant dryness (*Bryonia*, *Lycopodium*). There is neither a flakey skin complaint (*Sulphur*), nor constipation with hard, retained stools (*Alumina*, *Opium*, *Bryonia*, *Lycopodium*, *Plumbum met*).

This state of balance is one of constant adjustment as the key vital processes of body absorption, energy-extraction, drainage and excretion function during their 24 hour cycle. There is constant supply and distribution, where necessary, without interfering with the essential psychological processes of communication and thinking, both intuitive and logical, as the day moves through its inevitable 'ups and downs', successes and failures.

Energy reserves are built up for winter resistance in the spring, just as reserves for spring are accumulated six months before in the late summer. Man reflects the cosmos in the way he lays down patterns of vitality and health months before present resistance and reality, or sowing the seeds of disease by excess, denials and suppression, months

23

before an illness or breakdown occurs. An inadequate diet, or where aims and motivations are distorted or misplaced also leads to isolation from fundamental health-giving and universal principles.

The roots of a psychological illness can be seen months before an actual crisis occurs as a series of avoidances and self-negations which drain initiative and confidence from the functioning individuality at a cost to stability, resilience, balance and emotional health.

For many, the spring is the time when basic energy is liberated. There is a re-emergence of drive and initiative after a relatively fallow period of hibernation or inactivity. This is only partly stimulated by the morning dawn chorus, and physical factors – a rise in temperature, changes of green foliage or the emergence of brighter colours in the flowers – representing a shift in the bands of spectrum light-frequencies reflected upon the retina (Central Nervous System). All of these act as a natural stimulus to greater activity at this time. Spring remedies include *Crocus sat*, *Pulsatilla*, *Gelsemium*, *Arnica*, *Bellis perennis* (Daisy), *Ranunculus bulb* (Buttercup), with energy at a peak at this time. For others spring is a time for a low mood of depression and despair as the expectation of a magical cure for life's problems with the rising of the sap is not automatically forthcoming and life carries on as before. The long-awaited spontaneous cure can only occur when there is also a fundamental change in basic attitudes, priorities, initiative and less concern for self.

For some, the summer is their major time of fulfilment and action as the warmth of June and

July puts new life into them. Remedies especially associated with this time and most active are *Arsenicum*, *Calcarea*, *Apis*, *Sol*, *Calendula*, *Convallaria*, *Urtica*, *Formica*. In contrast, others are paralysed by heat developing problems of hay-fever, asthma, eczema, irritable indigestion, or rheumatism. *Kali carb* is a valuable remedy for summer problems and may help enormously with the 'allergic' catarrh, lethargy, rheumatic problems or chest spasm especially prevalent at the time, and often linked to high pollen counts. *Pulsatilla* is also of value where heat is paralysing.

Yet others have a late harvesting of energy flows and activity, like the bees bringing in a second, late nectar flow. *Colchicum*, *Aesculus hipp*, *Rhus tox*, *Dulcamara*, *Bryonia*, *Cyclamen* are good examples of autumn remedies. Mixed Autumn Pollen is another remedy used in the treatment of many allergic problems of mucus membrane that occur in the fall including rhinitis, conjunctivitis, late season hay-fever or asthma.

In winter it is natural to be quiet and for vital energy to be withdrawn deeply within the body as a protective instinct. Man lies fallow during the cold, inactive season and tends to attend only to life's basic necessities at a time for mulling over, thinking and planning. Homoeopathy takes account of this need for quiescence, to take stock, but notes the exceptions too and that some constitutions are at their best during a dry, bright cold spell especially *Sulphur*, *Pulsatilla*, *Argentum nitricum*. Other winter remedies include *Helleborus*, *Hamamelis*.

Illness occurs because of interference with

physiological or psychological processes leading to a build-up of toxic material or a depleted vitality. These impair resistance, so that sensitivity reactions are set up, which may be experienced as abnormal responses – for example to certain plants, to heat, cold, movement and effort. This sensitizing may occur in any area or situation where the initial cause or shock was overwhelming, leading to changed physiological or emotional responses and undermining the quality of life and spontaneity. When psychological sensitizing occurs, trust, closeness or confidence may be lost. With a physical condition, it may manifest as intolerance of certain common foods, to milk, gluten or the pollen of some grasses, flowers or trees, triggering-off an excessive response. A changed pattern of physiological functioning, impairs resistance, lowering vitality, concentration and drive.

The quality of life itself may be undermined or altered leading to a jaded sense of health or disease. Decision making and intellectual activity can be reduced, for example by severe hay-fever or chornic sinusitis. Trendy living, especially the fastfood habit, saps both nutrition and health, when not counteracted by a balanced diet. But especially the regular use of drugs, alcohol and tobacco, undermines the most robust constitutional health of adult or child sapping vitality and resistance. Their abuse causes premature aging even death, reinforcing problems of depression, anorexia and delinquency in a variety of forms.

Illness also occurs when there is an interference with natural patterns, as man becomes alienated from his birthright of instinct, spontaneity, intui-

tion and self-knowledge. In a stressful often con-
tracted, modern society, there is an increasing tendency to deny problems for reasons of anonymity
or withdrawal, and adults can close their eyes to
the needs of those most close to them, particularly
when these seem challenging, difficult or demanding. All of this leads to multiple difficulties and
complicated social problems in every age group,
even within the healthy family, unless there is open
communication, willingness to listen and discuss
the opinions and feelings of others, to understand
their realities and priorities and how the people
and personalities involved can best be helped.

Problems occur, because of natural differences
between every generation, the challenge of change
and an increasing tendency for people of every
creed, colour and background to be thrown
together without adequate preparation. This may
be either a very enriching experience, or a negative
one when there is refusal to express, to share,
support and relate with sufficient spontaneity,
tolerance and trust.

Increasingly, there is an unhealthy tendency for
ideas and values to be imposed by the political and
marketing media, undermining discrimination, and
identity, leading to strain, even confusion in some
cases. This same process is at work – not just in the
ways we think and perceive, but also how we eat
and what we choose and buy.

There is a tendency for foods to be in season
throughout the year and we no longer eat as our
ancestors did, according to the seasons and when
foods are most fresh and tasty. Additives, food
irradiation, processing and preservatives play a

sinister role to retain foodstuffs on the shelves for long periods, with a semblance of freshness far beyond their natural lifespan. All of this creates unnatural patterns without seasonal variation, impairing resistance and laying down the foundations for disease. The early Chinese philosophers, many centuries ago advocated only eating foods that were in season, preferably locally grown. But man is now largely alienated from such practical wisdom and philosophy – however homespun it may seem to some.

Just as we eat oranges all the year round – whether in season or not, so too we are expected to function in the same way, day after day, year after year, with little allowance given for individuality or need, the cycles of expansion and contraction, which involve us all to some extent. Increasingly attitudes become stereotyped, rigid or unbending with a tendency to perpetuate known familiar assumptions, whenever there is a challenge or a need for change. What is most needed for health and growth, is a set of new creative perspectives, related to each individual, to new experiences, to different ways of looking at problems, with greater understanding and a more overall experience of others.

In a similar way, the allotted fortnight in the sun may give too little time or energy for regeneration of new insights and understanding, for real contact with the local population, their culture, concerns and character. This can be a serious loss to individuality, depths, understanding, and one which could have contributed to a more expanded awareness and response which helps prevent illness. When this happens, the most mundane everyday situation is found to have a greater reality and meaning, a more meaningful perspective, leading to greater inner peace and tranquillity but especially to improved balance and health – even in a stressfull, media-dominated society.

Illness is the result of imbalance within the psyche or the physical body – often both. Where tensions exist, not fully dealt with at the time, then difficulties inevitably arise because there is an unresolved or neglected inner situation. Such a negative situation can quickly develop into a stress condition, leading to dis-ease and illness, or a chronic state of ill-health. Failure to deal with these personal realities at the time – perhaps a change in bowel pattern, or a psychological grief situation, may lead to chronic problems. Where there are unknowns and uncertainties as to causes and diagnosis, these can seem at the time to be a devastating challenge to our innate sense of immortality and provoke fear, depression or insecurity.

Unresolved tension areas may quickly become quite complicated psychological structures when neglected, as anxiety itself leads to a physical reponse of acidity, palpitations, hypertension, even diabetes, or joint and back pains. Loss of libido is also common. In extreme cases, the unresolved stress causes a heart attack or is a factor in the development of cancer, as retained emotions sink deeply into physical organs in an attempt to find a safe port for denial or a disguised alternative pathway of exit. At the same time however, they inevitably bring with them all their associated emotions which damage and undermine essential organ functioning.

In theory, such deep and profound outlets for stress, appear harmless, but delay in spontaneous expression puts quite basic physiological processes at risk and exposes vital organs to unnecessary pressures, and imbalance.

Every symptom is of interest and importance to the homoeopath because it reflects health and the strength of vital life-energies and with it the individuality of the person. The differences between individual responses is clearly shown by the wide variation of symptoms which occur and the modalities (or variation factors). An acute sore throat with a temperature is not an indication to prescribe an antibiotic for the homoeopath but the complaints indicate a particular remedy based on the symptom-pattern and appearance of the area affected. An acute throat, hot, red, and worse for swallowing indicates *Belladonna*. When the area is more white and dry, also aggravated by swallowing, this suggests *Bryonia*. A sensation in the throat of an irritating foreign body like a fish-bone, calls for *Hepar sulph*.; *Baryta carb* is indicated for an acute throat with marked lymph gland involvement and tenderness; *Phytolacca* is for painful tonsillitus with a purple discolouration. *Silicea* is prescribed where there is painful swelling and a discharge of pus; *Sulphur* may be needed where the throat condition is particularly offensive; *Rhus tox* is for a milder condition, and better for swallowing; *Diptherinum* is indicated for the most acute difficulties with a web on the tonsil and near-paralysis of the swallowing mechanism.

But to some degree, every illness begins with some disturbance within the deepest most central core of the person, namely the mind or psyche, where an unexpressed response or area of feeling leads to the accumulation of negative patterns and attitudes. There may be excessive concern with being right or wrong, with winning, rather than playing the game of life, or of just being. There is usually extreme over-intensity or competitiveness to the detriment of relaxed individuality and easy self-expression, undermining relationships generally. Such a disturbance is reflected externally by anxiety symptoms. These include palpitations (*Spigelia*), sweating (*Silicea*), nausea (*Ipecuanha*), physical insecurity (*Argentum nit.*), or social discomfort (*Natrum mur.*). Internally they may be felt as panic (*Lycopodium*), fear (*Aconitum*), tension (*Nux. vomica*). Depression, irritability and lack of energy are other common expressions. The deepest most central aspect of man's being is undoubtedly the spiritual core. When this is affected, with psychological depletion, there is frequently a deep crisis of faith with loss of belief and trust in an overall pattern or meaning to life. This gives added despair to the common feelings of isolation and loneliness.

Symptoms are the essential key to prescribing and the basis of every homoeopathic prescription, determined by matching the patient's overall 'problem-picture' to the profile of the remedies. Often the individual's life-style has become distorted beyond recognition. An unnatural compromise between aims, and ideals, principles, and beliefs may have developed, because of financial or

31

just day to day pressures. All too often, true to Parkinson's Law – the more we have the more we want, creates an unending spiral which leads to chronic malaise and ill-health. Such life-styles bring conflicts with unbearable frustrations. The psychologically and environmentally alienated lives, remote from any true self, real motivations or need, creates psychological havoc, spiritual devastation and emptiness, expending precious irreplaceable reserves of life and energy.

Under such circumstances, demands and pressures, any natural balance is quickly lost and problems of tension, fatigue, constipation and insomnia occur – even in the young. For many, the underlying dissatisfactions are a cry for help, as life becomes so complicated that no longer does the dog wag the tail, but the tail the dog, and by any measure of vitality and health, this is a recipe for disaster.

Each symptom says something about the individual concerned as well as the site of irritation and degree of damage. In homoeopathy every symptom is assessed and evaluated according to individuality and a remedy chosen which most closely matches the individual needs with the remedy's ability to act at a site of vitality depletion, to support energy flow and reinstate functioning where this is possible. When there is more persistent damage or irreversible tissue changes, as from a severe burn, motorway or industrial accident, then a conventional approach using surgery, fluid replacement and skin grafting may be required.

Excessive exposure to the sun may cause severe burning or blistering (*Cantharis*, *Apis*, *Urtica*) as many know to their discomfort and when exposure is severe or prolonged, serious (second-degree) burns can occur. Skin cancer (*Sol*, *X-ray*) may be the result of prolonged exposure over the years, although it is increasingly seen in young men or women, possibly linked to the vogue for an artificial tan and the use of sunbeds. But at the same time, all symptoms reflect a positive attempt by the organism to re-establish order and vitality within the physiological configurations of the individual and to maintain homoeostasis or a healthy overall balance.

In homoeopathy, an initial aggravation or worsening of symptoms following the remedy, often indicates a positive change in underlying patterns and anticipates a return to health in the area being treated. Where the origins of a condition are denied, obscure or unconscious, the patient's own role in his illness not admitted, then homoeopathy may be more difficult to prescribe, but it can still be curative, as long as the symptom-profile has been accurately observed and the correct remedy and potency given.

Only in extreme or terminal cases, or where there is unbearable physical pain should symptoms be deliberately suppressed. This avoids a pathological process being pushed deeper into more remote areas which are difficult for the vital processes to reach and heal. Increasingly organ tension is becoming more commonplace and an everyday medical problem. Diabetes, asthma, colitis, hypertension, thyrotoxicosis, reflect pressurised modern man with accumulations of unresolved tone and energy thrust into physiological processes where they undermine functioning and are difficult for the body to eliminate.

Symptoms vary with each individual whatever the genetic make up. Everyone has their own unique way of reacting and responding to the demands and pressures that daily occur as the body attempts to restore equilibrium or to neutralise adverse reactions without harmful denial or suppression.

But even the most negative symptom has its positive side and an apparently harmful symptom of chest wheezing or tightness can be a powerful attempt to expel a mucus plug or stimulate oxygenation of the lung tissues. In depressive illness, there are similar positive attempts to expel a sense of failure or feelings of futility, bringing unconscious feelings nearer to the surface, makes them more available for awareness and insight. In this way every illness – even a psychological one has its positive side and reflects quite powerful moves to restore confidence, balance and health.

Case reports

A woman aged 32 came recently with a recurrence of genital herpes. She was confident that the condition was aggravated by recent examination anxieties and the breakdown in the relationship with her boyfriend (*Natrum mur*).

A man of 78 came with recurrent prostatic difficulties. He was positive that the recent aggravation of urinary problems was because of business 'pressures' – especially the need for redundancies in staff who had served him faithfully over many years.

Every symptom is a healthy response to pressures and stress of some kind and a reaction to them as the body attempts to correct the imbalance. Such symptom expressions are important reactions to be conserved and fostered by the homoeopathic approach rather than something to be eradicated or suppressed because they are inconvenient. Energy and reserves are needed to create a symptom however much a contradiction this may seem, reflecting healthy reactive functioning and positive drives toward health and healing.

For the majority, symptoms are a very intimate and personal expression of the individual. The child with a tendency to be quick and impatient, may be equally acute and rapid in his pattern of illnesses, quickly ill with pain and a high temperature but equally well and responding rapidly to the homoeopathic approach. Another of the same family may be more sluggish to develop a fever and generally slow in all things, with a tendency to hold back, slow to reveal himself. A pattern of illness which is drawn-out takes longer to treat and cure. The overall tendency to sluggish reactions, passivity of growth and thinking holds true for the way that body-symptoms develop and is an aspect of the overall personality. These patterns of responding and of individuality, are often highlighted during a physical illness.

CHAPTER FOUR

The basic causation of illness and disease

Whatever the precise trigger factor or precipitating cause, all illness is ultimately the expression of a combination of multiple factors, including external pressures and internal psychological change. The roots of disease lie in the deepest part of the person – a constitutional or genetic predisposition to organ weakness or psychological self-destructive attitudes. Normal balanced physiological functioning is dependent upon a healthy interaction between constitutional, genetic (miasmic), physical and psychological areas.

In illness there is a lack of liaison between the two great fundamentals and imbalance or disease is the outcome. When an individual is psychologically depleted by underlying anxiety, depressive problems, or stress of any kind, then this has a draining effect and is debilitating to energy supplies and body functioning. Particularly digestive functioning is interfered with, so that the break-down of energy-providers or foods is lessened to the body's reserves. At the same time, the excretory channels of the bowel become less efficient, with all the discomfort of toxic-reabsorption, stasis, infection, and constipation.

In a similar way, when there is an external or physical problem, for example – varicose veins, recurrent sinusitis, or chronic catarrh, this affects the underlying confidence, poise and attitudes generally, as drive is sapped by the disturbance.

In every case, whenever the underlying psychological state is interfered with, by feelings or emotions that cannot adequately or easily be contained, this depletes energy and natural resistance, paving the way for illness.

The following are often instrumental – directly or indirectly, in the development of disease and are usually explored during the initial and subsequent homeopathic consultations in a search to understand the precipitating causes and overall meaning of an illness.

Inherited factors

These are the areas of inherited achilles heel or constitutional flaw, which we all have to some extent. Adler called them areas of 'organ weakness' which run through families, giving a tendency to skin problems, chest weakness, infection in certain parts of the body and sometimes migraine attacks. The problem is an inherited one, but different from the more obvious chromosomal and predictable transmitted diseases as haemophilia, because the links are more subtle and tenuous.

37

Homoeopathy calls these inherited tendencies –
the Miasms.

Case reports

An example occurred recently with a colleague.
She developed a worrying problem of an irritating
summer dry cough which was very troublesome
and tended to recur year after year for no apparent
cause. There was a strong history of tuberculosis in
the family which had affected several members
over more than one generation, although she had
never been directly involved in any way with the
disease. Exhaustive tests had always been completely negative. When the nosode of the tuberculosis illness – *Tuberculinum* was given, she made
a rapid recovery from all the symptoms whereas
conventional medicine had consistently failed to
evoke any curative response whatsoever. We can
assume that this was the typical tuberculosis miasm
at work and controlled by its nosode or
homoeopathic vaccine. My colleague needed the
Tuberculinum yearly to control the symptoms
which recurred less acutely for three years. She has
not required the nosode since. At the age of eight-
een, her daughter developed similar symptoms
which also responded quickly to the same nosode
prescription.

Another example of inherited factors at work
and causing disease occurred in identical twins.
One brother needed help for a chronic prostate
problem, the other had a back problem. Both were
aged 65. Most striking was that each developed a
right-sided hernia or rupture, needing surgery,

within weeks of the other at a time when they were living many miles apart and unaware that the other had a similar weakness.

Identical twins, in spite of chromosomal similarities always show considerable variation in energy availability and symptom patterns although they may look physically alike. One twin had a long history of recurrent depressive breakdowns, inability to cope and periods of hospitalisation, with a passive personality preferring the 'quiet approach', but feeling inadequate and a little too easy-going and unsure of herself. The other twin in complete contrast, was aggressive, noisy, assertive and full of confidence. Bossy and organising, she always had something to say, was too free with her advice and a complete psychological opposite to her sister (*Platina*).

In another pair of twins, in their eighties, one had chronic bowel problems, with incapacitating indigestion, distension and flatulence, (*Carbo veg*, *Lycopodium*, *Argentum nit*), and a passive, quiet temperament. Her sister and mirror-image had never seen a day's illness in her life. She was constitutionally strong and confident without any of the problems of self-doubt and anguish which plagued her sister.

Inheritance plays a role in such diverse diseases as cancer, heart disease, diabetes, hypertension, psoriasis and hay fever. In some, the full illness does not develop, and there may be only mild symptoms at times of stress, hormonal imbalance or environmental pressure. A combination of emotional strain, high pollen count, exhaustion and fatigue may provoke symptoms which would not

39

usually be present at 'normal' times.

In others, no obvious or direct inherited link is known, yet there is weakness and vague symptoms in one particular area. The suspicion of a hereditary weakness or miasm may make it inadvisable to smoke, use the 'Pill' or be prescribed hormonal replacements when there is a family history of heart disease, circulatory weakness, or sometimes cancer.

Exhaustion

Weakness may occur, and a homoeopathic remedy be indicated when there has been a period of exhausting physical or psychological wear and tear over a prolonged period as the vitality batteries are run down.

Fatigue is common after a period of excessive devotion to duty, as the prolonged nursing of a sick relative or friend over weeks or months takes its toll. For depleted reserves, *China* is often invaluable, with *Arnica*, *Nux moschata*, *Arsenicum*, *Kali carb* alternatives to consider.

It is quite usual to find underlying feelings of psychological resentment present and sometimes guilt is involved which adds to the fatigue. A relative is often difficult or demanding and there may be many mixed feelings about the necessity of a nursing-home admission. Usually a lot of tension is present which adds to the physical load leaving a sense of exhaustion and insomnia despite the fatigue. A depressive breakdown may occur unless prevented in time by good sense and at least some relief from the physical burden.

In others exhaustion occurs after a particularly severe or prolonged physical effort – a cross-country race in a nervous adolescent who is not fit, particularly where finishing well and status are the priorities. Similar problems can also occur in the elderly – after pneumonia or bronchitis, with fatigue on climbing stairs, also from failing lung and cardiac functioning – the least effort a strain and a demand (*China*, *Phosphorus*, *Nux moschata*, *Convallaria*, *Crataegus*, *Phosphoric acid*).

Exhaustion may also be the result of atmospheric pollution particularly from toxic car fumes, high levels of lead (*plumbum met*) or carbon monoxide. Other considerations are a general lack of fresh air and exercise to stimulate circulation and healthy lung activity. An inadequate diet, too low in protein, carbohydrates, minerals or vitamins may be another factor in third world countries.

But for many, over-eating and obesity are far more important than dietary deficiency. Stagnation from protein intoxication and the accumulation of body lipids (fats) in the organs and blood vessels is a major danger and threat to health. Most important of all is the psychological health of each individual taking priority over the factors mentioned, even the inherited ones. Where there is psychological imbalance, unresolved pressure or stress, or restraint upon spontaneity, then these inevitably take their toll on the vital energy reserves. Their depletion is a major cause of loss of interest, exhaustion, lack of drive and expression.

Allergic factors

The commonest allergic factors seen are hay-fever, eczema and asthma, although at times non-specific conditions occur with generalised swelling of the face and fingers or whole body after certain foods, especially those containing gluten or on exposure to a dusty environment. Allergic triggers are typically pollen, house-dust, cat and animal hair, certain foods, dairy products, particularly cow's milk (*Aethusa*) with allergy developing in the infant when breast-feeding, as the allergen is transmitted across the natural barrier of mother to child and becomes present in the milk. The attacks are always rather paradoxical and unpredictable, with no known definite pattern, varying with each social situation as much as the pollen count. There is nearly always a lot of anticipation and fear when the attacks occur. In many cases, a powerful psychological element is undoubtedly at work as well as a more straight-forward allergic one. For many patients, however strict the desensitizing diet or injections, they are ineffective because they do not take into account the full depth of the problem.

Psychological factors

The emotions are an important major cause of illness in at least a third to a half of all patients in the general surgery and in some areas the figures are as high as 75% of those seen. Shock, rejection, stress of any kind, misunderstanding, rivalry problems, competition, jealousy – not adequately dealt with and talked through at the time – may provoke in the sensitive, imperative strong feelings which are also felt to be unacceptable or a cause of guilt. For some, whenever there is a pressure or demand, an unexpected change, crisis at work – having to lay-off workers who have been loyal over the years – this creates an intolerable situation of turmoil and anguish. When such emotional realities are not faced up to, because the changes or decisions conflict with life-long patterns, even principles, then a conflict arises which becomes attached to the more acceptable physical processes. Change, however essential for economic or personal survival, may be bitterly resented and often there are unconscious attempts to delay a painful reality which cannot be faced up to. When feelings of this kind are suppressed, not shared or talked about, nor given expression in some way, they are inevitably driven deeply, only to re-emerge as feelings of guilt, depression, inadequacy, collapse or panic. A negative inner energy sphere may be formed without an outlet which can lead to severe mental illness if left unresolved and untreated.

Shock, rejection, anger, misunderstanding, rivalry, competition and jealousy may all provoke severe feelings which at the time are felt to be uncontrollable. These feelings *need* to be expressed and given life in order to be reasonably satisfied and dealt with at the time and to avoid the canker of underlying resentment developing its inherent destructiveness. Avoidance of psychological conversion-symptoms is important, as when these occur they take with them a great deal of the energy and drive belonging to their original problem when re-sited, in what is usually an inappropri-

43

ate physical area. When this happens in the chest it may provoke asthma or chronic bronchitis, within the bowels it can cause colitis, and when the skin is used to contain emotion, psoriasis or an eczema problem may occur. Excessive emotional tension in the duodenum or alimentary tract may result in duodenal ulceration. These physical developments, do nothing to relieve or resolve the underlying psychological basic hurt and only further complicate life because there is the added worry of an often dangerous physical problem draining vitality and the healthy functioning of the organ(s) involved.

Epidemic factors

At times, and frequently where preventative hygiene has become non-existent, certain diseases of viral or bacterial origin expand and develop. They are often insect or animal-carried and create multiple attacks within a large area so that epidemics occur. The exact cause may not be clearly known and often a new strain of bacteria or virus appears, resistant to all known antibiotics. This can devastate the health of thousands, particularly the elderly, although illness may occur at any age.

Influenza was a particularly severe problem in the winter of 1985–86 and again in the late spring, when in the UK thousands were affected with either gastric influenza as severe watery diarrhoea with exhaustion (*Arsenicum*, *Influenzinum*) or chest problems, as bronchitis or pneumonia (*Influenzinum*, *Tub. bov.*, *Bryonia*, *Phosphorus*).

There were many deaths amongst the elderly from viral pneumonia especially when reserves and

44

resistance fell to a fatal low due to toxic reactions from the virus. Other common epidemic illnesses still seen are poliomyelitis (endemic in many third world countries); diptheria (an epidemic occurred in Goteburg, Sweden in 1985); typhoid (endemic in many countries), meningitis (endemic in the UK, for nearly a decade in parts of Gloucestershire). Psychological illnesses can also take an epidemic turn as occurred in Israel in 1985 (hysteria). But on the whole epidemics are usually physical in type, infective in origin and spread by contact, usually from lack of hygiene or where there is overcrowding. As a result of global air transport almost any disease can suddenly develop epidemic proportions, especially in poor ghetto areas, indeed anywhere where there is poverty and poor standards of nutrition.

Mechnical factors

When there is interference to normal physiological functioning from any cause – displacement, non-alignment of the spine, injury or blockage, leads to narrowing of normal channels and interference with elimination, absorption and drainage causing pain and discomfort. Physical damage from the trauma of a traffic accident, chronic ulceration or the breakdown of a wound after surgery, comes into this category because of the formation of scar-tissue which at a later date may contract and cause distortion of neighbouring tissues.

Traumatic displacement of the cervical (neck) region, involving the spinal ligaments, commonly follows a whiplash injury. Other mechanical causes of stiffness and pain are dislocation, congenital deformations – for example divided or absent spinal processes (spina bifida), congenital cysts of the kidney, intestine or bladder – which require surgical correction. Damage to ligaments is common after a precipitate childbirth causing uterine prolapse or chronic pelvic and bladder problems. Digestive or intestinal malfunctioning may be due to spasm and imbalance within the organs concerned or to irritation of the spinal nerve segments leading to spasm, acidity and ulceration. Depending upon the cause, surgical repair, spinal manipulation or physiotherapy are required in addition to any specific homoeopathic treatment.

Other causes of mechanical blockage and pain are hernia, local pressure from a boil, abscess, cyst, fatty swelling or tumour pushing and pressing on neighbouring nerve tissues causing numbness or shooting pains in the area (*Hypericum*). Pain from an arthritic condition of the knee or hip, or following an operation for joint replacement may also cause limitation of movement. Symptoms are not always felt in the area affected. Pain from a hip abnormality is often experienced at the knee. Irritation of the diaphragm is commonly experienced at the shoulder, a deep peptic ulcer may give pain between the shoulder blades. A bladder or prostate problem can cause discomfort along the thigh region to the knee.

Homoeopathy treats symptoms as well as their cause whenever possible. Other mechanical conditions where homoeopathy plays a secondary role are chest pain from a pacemaker, not seated satisfactorily within the pectoral tissues; uterine irritation from an IUD; a club foot dating back to an illness in early pregnancy or abnormal uterine position; recurrent dislocation (*Calcarea*). All of these need some physical correction before homoeopathy is fully effective.

Parasitic factors

These are important in certain tropical countries where invasion of bowel and surrounding tissues by tape, round and thread worms is endemic. Round worms, hydatid cysts and bilharzia are seen in many middle Eastern and tropical countries and have become much more widely seen with the age of rapid jet-travel to all parts of the world. They are a constant factor to be considered whenever chronic disease is not responding to the usual measures.

Parasitic disease has become increasingly common in this country and it is now common to see parents as well as childern troubled by anal irritation at night due to thread worms. General restlessness and irritation are a feature, with facial ticks, grimacing, teeth grinding or nasal itching. Insomnia is also common with problems of sleepwalking, general restlessness or dreams and nightmares. *Cina* is one of the best remedies for the condition but as always in homoeopathy it is the symptoms that dictate the remedy and not the diagnostic label in isolation from the individual. Other useful remedies include *Santonin*, and *Teucrium*. Where Ringworm is a problem, *Sepia* or *Tellurium* should be considered.

47

Poisoning factors

These are on the increase with dust lead levels now at a peak in many of our cities and carbon monoxide at times beyond the safety limit. Babies and young children are especially vulnerable to these environmental toxic factors especially atmospheric lead, (*Plumbum*). Although this has been largely eradicated from paint and toys, the levels of air pollution in our high density urban areas are a major cause for concern. Mercury (*Mercurius*) is increasingly found in water because of spillage from industrial sprays and agricultural herbicides – it is exceedingly toxic and at least as dangerous as lead. Pharmacological poisoning now occurs with many drugs widely used in the home especially aspirin, antihistamines or sedatives. In excess they undermine health and well-being especially when taken regularly over a long period for reasons of dependency.

Iatrogenic factors (doctor-induced illness)

There is little doubt that the side-effects and complications of modern allopathic medicines is one of the major factors in patient-complaints and illness of our time. Drug-induced illness or drug dependency is now a major problem in every surgery throughout the country and the number of patients who are addicted to sedatives, tranquillizers, purgatives, anti-depressants and pain-killers runs into millions and probably tens of millions if the European population is considered and the pattern of prescriptions looked at more closely.

There are many who had no psychological illness of addiction or dependency initially, but having started a course of treatment and become more or less free from symptoms, they are quite unable to give up the medicines from fear of a relapse. They still feel insecure and that they 'need' to take something to remain well. Withdrawal of these drugs is impossible in a busy surgery because of the time required to explore each individual's anxieties.

When this occurs, the tendency is not to stop the treatment and to observe the patient, but to switch to a similar related drug in the vain hope that no new reactions will be forthcoming. But dependency patterns are now increasingly accepted as 'normal' and no longer a response-of-disease or abnormal psychological response.

The anti-depressants, blood-pressure (hypotensive drugs), contraceptive 'pill', and hormone therapies, together with the steroid group of suppressants are the major culprits.

Their action, outside the therapeutically desired one is often too broad-ranging, involving the heart and circulation, immune defensive system, and vital organs of the livery and kidneys, which may all be affected by a variety of side-effects and dysfunction. The remedies, although important and of value, when over-prescribed provoke the very same symptoms which they are trying to cure and can serve to reinforce an original illness. This has been clearly shown to occur with certain tranquillizers, prescribed by the billion, which cause symptoms of tension and anxiety in their own right. Even the vital anti-spasmodics used for asthma

49

have been shown to provoke bronchial spasm when there is an allergic reaction to the synthetic colorants used in pill-coatings.

Socially-induced factors

These factors are the other illnesses of addiction, now so commonplace and subtle in many cases as to be accepted as normal, but where the symptoms and the health repercussions are enormously important for the overall well being and vitality of the person. I am thinking here of such social-addictions and government-revenue earners as cigarettes and alcohol as causes of disease. The former, has a proven action (of tobacco) on the lungs, heart and circulation, which also stunts growth of the young foetus. There is a much smaller placenta, umbilical cord and birth weight and often chest problems in the neonate. There are further grave implications for cancer of adults and circulatory disease for every young woman on the 'pill'. Despite the warning notices, in general the public has not been fully advised of the true dangers and only a minimum has been done to put over clearly that these are potential killers. In spite of this the advertising goes on and more and more young people still use cigarettes or their attractive packaging as a social-prop and symbol of their new-found maturity.

Alcohol is another one of the major disease-inducers of our time, a poison to the delicate cells of the liver, heart and brain when regularly taken in excess. I am not referring here to the often advantageous tonic action of social drinking or wine in moderation with meals.

I still see lonely, isolated people, men and women, from a wide variety of social backgrounds, often of mature years who drink regularly to obliterate or forget. Depressed and lonely, usually feeling hopeless, they rarely eat adequately at mealtimes and with each successive bottle taken, become more and more trapped, unhappy and down. Unable to find or go for help or advice, they slowly destroy themselves both physically and psychologically.

The other common social diseases are those caused by excess of coffee, tea or sugar, all of which are addictive and undesirable, causing either hypoglycaemia, vitality-collapse, restlessness or nervous tension. All caffeine-containing drinks may affect quite fundamental areas of a person's physiology, including the menstrual cycle. The role in disease of the dubious, but widespread practice of using additives, colorants, preservatives, stabilisers, oxidisers, artificial flavour and sweetener agents in basic foods is still uncertain. Many have been withdrawn because of their association with possible cancer-formations and fortunately they are now under more constant scrutiny. Doubtless we are not yet at the end of the list of those due for withdrawal and their whole purpose – to artificially prolong storage and shelf-life and to give an apparent freshness – is highly questionable. Even the so-called 'harvest-foods' too often contains additives if the labels are scrutinized. Their role in disease formation is one to be constantly on the watch for in the press. Be prepared to discard any suspect food should warning be given.

Many jobs are associated with illness, especially where there has been insufficient knowledge or research carried out to prevent toxicity from the basic materials used. For example, Asbestosis is common in those who work with asbestos in brake-linings, paint and post-office line workers causing sterility, impotency and chronic lung disease. There is a higher incidence of cancer in radiographers. Addiction to sedatives, stimulants and amphetamines is common in doctors and nurses because of the easy availability and access or they have been routinely prescribed over the years for slimming, depression or exhaustion. Bronchitis and emphysema tend to be more common in miners, transport drivers and car park attendants where levels of lead in the dust and atmosphere and carbon monoxide fumes are still unacceptably high.

An elderly widow, now living alone, may have to carry heavy shopping bags and as a result develops uterine prolapse or varicose veins. Sometimes the underlying despair and depression is expressed more psychologically as shop-lifting in a desperate attempt to gain attention or help. The need to make pills more attractive and colourful produces other problems. As with colourants in food a variety of allergic reactions may develop as a sensitivity-response, ranging from eczema to the more serious problem of asthma. Where a known colourant has been identified as causing symptoms – it should be avoided. If this is not possible, then the colourant in potency may be made up by a homoeopathic pharmacist and used as a specific

52

remedy to resolve the problem.

Media influence, particularly television has an effect on freedom of choice and behaviour, especially where there is a too ready acceptance of violence by the family without comment. Being aggressive has now become a symbol of what is modern and tough having a negative effect on many immature, impressionable youngsters, especially when combined with the widely available stimulant drugs – glues, heroin, cannabis, marijuana, cocaine. It is not surprising that social patterns and values are undermined and that violence in young people has become a global issue.

Media advertising encourages both alcohol intake and cigarette smoking. It is still too often linked to a sporty, virile success image by the advertisers. A major contribution to the present social malaise, is the passive attitude of many parents to behaviour problems in their children. They are often confused as to how to act, discuss and discipline, fearing firmness or having any controls or rules is old-fashioned yet finding that permissiveness does little either to foster communication or respect within the family.

In education, many teachers now find that they have a major discipline problem in their classes which undermines their essential educational role, with often too little backing from the top. Firmness rules and punishment can lead to dismissal or violence from a pupil or his family. In the pupil it is too often condoned as youthful exuberance or a positive expression, but for teachers to control or punish has become unpardonable. The same problem is now developing in hospitals and casualty departments where violence is increasingly common. With fewer controls or deterrents, a background of fast food, fast music and television programmes which idealise violence, it is not surprising that social malaise is on the increase and a major backcloth to much of the physical and psychological illness which is undermining society.

Dietary factors

Most people still eat a poorly balanced meal, far too rich in starches, sugars and animal protein for their adult needs. It is often lacking in essential fibre-content, natural vitamins, minerals and adequate raw-food as vegetables and fresh fruit. This is especially true for the elderly but also for teenagers. The former live alone, neglecting themselves, because it is difficult to cook and buy for one and a bun and jam is easiest to make, especially a frozen or pre-cooked one. The teenager wants hamburgers, chips, coke and a sweet milkshake because their taste-buds are formed by the media and not by nutritional requirements or vitality-needs.

During homoeopathic treatment, it is important to avoid all strong stimulants – spices and herbs such as ginger, curry, peppermint, menthol, chamomile, tea or coffee. The intake of cigarettes and alcohol should be kept to a sensible minimum or avoided altogether to allow the remedies to act with as little external interference as possible. Meals should be simple, regular, well-chewed and light, during treatment. A high-fibre diet assists elimination and is recommended unless wheat bran is a factor in gluten sensitivity or causes flatulence, when soya-bran may be substituted.

In general, food should be eaten as fresh as possible, organically grown and unsprayed. It must be thoroughly washed before use and then only lightly cooked or steamed for a minimum of time to retain flavour, essential vitamins and minerals. Aluminium utensils should not be used in cooking as they are toxic when used with acid fruits. Where cirrhosis or gout is a problem, alcohol, game and rich foods should be strictly forbidden. If there is a heart problem, history of heart disease, or where blood pressure increased, then foods rich in saturated fats as red meat, dairy products, avocado, coconut, eggs, saturated cooking oils should be avoided and smoking should be banned.

Frozen food, heated in the microwave is not nutritionally ideal for the homoeopathic patient either and more simple good food is recommended. Where eating habits are not regular, nor associated with a feeling of peace, appreciation and reverence, then meals should be small as chronic indigestion lays a strong foundation for disease. The combination of indequate rest, excess weight, lack of exercise and no peace of mind has all the ingredients for disease and illness. A balanced mind, rhythmic life with worry and strain kept minimal and problems dealt with and verbalised as they occur, is the simplest and best approach to the prevention of disease.

Stress factors

Distinct from the psychological factors outlined, this section could equally be called diseases of modern living or modern times. Here illness is caused by the more subtle indefinable factors of constant pressure, wear-and-tear, rush, lack of rhythm, noise and pace generally. The general philosophy underlying stress is the assumption that 'time is money' or 'a minute gained is a minute saved'. But if you ask what has been done with the minutes saved, the reply is vague and negative. Discord, lack of balance, purposeless competitive drives, all take their toll psychologically and physiologically with tension and pain across the shoulders, low-back, elbows and shoulders. Fibrositis, rheumatism, indigestion, constipation, high blood-pressure, strokes, peptic ulcer and gall-bladder disease are but few of the social diseases of our time and civilisation. They are all common, their exact cause from a variety of pressures and stresses with poor dietary intake and psychological factors combining to undermine vitality and allow the development of disease and premature degenerative changes.

Environmental factors

These factors are now common in all parts of the world. For many people, crowded, inadequately heated offices, poorly illuminated workshops, with no natural daylight are the norm. Open-plan offices create an environment of being surrounded by too many people in a large noisy and smokey impersonal space with little privacy, creating depression and undermining health. Over-heating is a negative factor in most modern offices or homes causing a dry atmosphere, after the stress and tension of commuting to the office under pressurised conditions. It is not surprising that many young people are already tired before their day begins. The result is that heart-attacks are now occurring in both men and women at an increasingly young age. Nervous breakdowns, the addictions discussed, obesity, or its counterpart anorexia are also seen frequently.

At the end of the day there is an unhealthy, jaded sense of fatigue and collapse. Some are too tired to eat properly and another snack-meal is the common pattern. More and more people are leading mindless, passive lives glued to the television or isolated under headphones. They are often full of good intentions but too exhausted and tired to carry them through into reality. The pressures are eventually translated into physical change, recognizable disease and symptoms in one form or another. Prevention by early diagnosis should be the first priority and the patient treated well before physical and irreversible cellular changes occur. Many run the gauntlet of conventional treatments before homoeopathy is given a trial – not infrequently in desperation or as a last resort – rather than as a first line of safe effective treatment.

As technology gallops ahead of the people using it for commercial, competitive or political reasons, there is a minimum of controls, sound research and environmental concern. It is inevitable that disasters occur and Chernobyl is only one example of this. In every country, there is now global pollution with radio-active Iodine, Strontium and Cesium. DDT is also globally distributed. Nuclear reactor leaks are becoming regular happenings in many countries – the UK, France, Scandinavia, Russia

57

and USA, to name but a few. The level of child leukaemia incidence in these nuclear reactor zones is also worryingly high and the true mortality from industrial leakages is still not exactly known, nor disclosed.

Low-frequency hum, dust and industrial vibration are other factors which undermine health and well-being in our industrialised society and are an unrecognized hazard to the population. They cause various syndromes and problems which are only just beginning to be known about. Homoeopathy can play a specific major role in their treatment, once the causes are clarified.

CHAPTER FIVE

The indications for Homoeopathy

For convenience these have been grouped into acute and chronic problems, but there are really no fixed or firm dividing lines where people are concerned and each problem must be dealt with on merit according to the severity of the problem and individual make-up.

Acute Problems

Psychological

Because of its unique action in the mental sphere, homoeopathy has a major role to play in the treatment of emotional and psychological problems. Recent figures estimate for the UK approximately 15 million cases of depression in treatment and there are at least as many of anxiety-tension. It is likely too that these figures are on the low side. About one case in three seen in the surgery has a weighted psychological element to it when the symptoms are not clearly emotional from the start. Common problems, where homoeopathy plays a useful role, include phobias of all types where the predominant emotion is fear (*Aconitum, Arg. nit*); tension states where there is an excess of keyed-up emotion (*Natrum mur*) and fixed illogical states of mind not amenable to reason – often of an obsessional type. (*Stramonium*, *Nux vom*, Thuja, *Belladonna*). Homoeopathy can help in all of these conditions, depending on the length and severity of the problem. Particularly the high potencies of 200C upwards are helpful because they resonate at these depths within the psyche.

Homoeopathy assists by re-aligning displaced psychological processes, putting them back into balance, much as it will help a displaced physical condition which does not require mechanical correction. It assists in the easing and freeing of rigid patterns of thinking and perception which otherwise form barriers and knots to closeness, relationships, understanding and perception of the world as it is, rather than as it is imagined to be. Fixed assumption patterns, like sullen anger, hard attitudes, hurts and resentments die slowly unless they are brought out into the open and looked at with mature eyes to soften and see them also as valuable parts of life's overall mosaic.

Homoeopathy helps release and unlock pent up over-intense areas, where energy and drive is attached and expressed through physical channels – the heart as palpitations, large intestine as colitis, the stomach as acidity, flatulence or spasm. Such expressions and exits can become a worrying chronic problem when they occur over months or years. The individual may often be best helped or a problem mobilised, by a constitutional remedy followed by a specific local treatment. Once talked about, preoccupation with the past can be softened, with less domination by imagined hurts, the energy and happenings of the present allowed more say within an overall self-expression in the fullness of the present.

The specific trigger to a psychological problem is often the combination of a physical situation and a contemporary stress or pressure.

Common casebook examples are – a fall on the ice at a skating-rink during adolescence – at a time of anxiety about a change of schools next term, or the parents in marital crisis. A fall at the time, even though causing only minor bruising, can nevertheless fix and crystalise much of the emotional flow into recurrent headaches or neck stiffness. In a sensitive girl these may become increasingly difficult to treat with the passing of time. With another personality the outcome might have been phobic or clinging, regressive demanding infantile behaviour breaking into adult maturity. This can create a vicious circle of 'nobody cares' or 'nobody loves me' leading to depression.

Other psychological areas commonly helped by homoeopathy are the psycho-sexual difficulties – lack of confidence with the opposite sex, frigidity, impotence (*Agnus cast*, *Lycopodium*), spasm (*Tabacum*) premature ejaculation (*Lycopodium*), lack of interest (*Sepia*). Often the pattern of what seems an obvious sexual problem is in fact only one frame or image of an overall constitutional disturbance, where frigidity or premature explosive attitudes dominate most other forms of expression. There is commonly a short-fuse reaction in dealing with any confrontation or situation where a degree of holding back and pacing of the self is required and the sexual problem is only a relatively minor aspect of far broader disturbances.

It is here that individual constitutional prescribing is valuable because of its overall action, promoting relaxation and spontaneity. Improvement can occur in these personal areas – wrongly felt as a demand to perform – as the pressures are reduced. This helps put the sexual act and other areas of personal expression more into perspective – in itself therapeutic.

Marital stress is another common area where homoeopathy is helpful. It can play an important role, especially where infantile demands and expectations have displaced more solid caring, sensitive feelings, (*Pulsatilla*, *Calcarea*, *Baryta carb*). The right homoeopathic remedy backed by a consultation which explores the reasons why immature attitudes dominate mature sensitivity, may tip the balance in favour of seeing the partner more as a person, rather than as an off-shoot of a feared or fantasised internal object. Roles and labels have usually been ascribed over months or years and homoeopathy by its freeing action supports new dialogue and more balanced mature attitudes, giving the opportunity for tangible change and growth to occur within the couple.

Often both members need to be seen at some time and treated constitutionally. This not only helps the relationship, but also avoids a situation where only one is seen as ill or sick, needing treatment and the other as cooperative and healthy. Such divisions and splits prolong or even confirm unhealthy attitudes which undermine the fundamentals of the relationship.

Where there is an actual mental illness or break with reality, a retreat into an unreal world of fantasy and psychosis, then inevitably the problem needs more specialised help. Treatment with high potency remedies may be needed over a period of months. Illness of this type can be a long drawn-out matter, especially where the psychotic process is in the ascendance, distorting body and mind of any reality to obliterate the experience of being, knowing and feeling. For the psychotic mind, existence and awareness are only associated with one thing – a combination of hurt, rejection, control or interference, but especially pain. Homoeopathy helps build-up the more positive residual elements of the ego, which are always present and once these cohere, and become more stable and secure they underpin often weaker areas of fragility and vulnerability which constantly threaten health by an emotional landslide.

A combination of homoeopathy, experience, consistent support, understanding, sympathetic therapy, with hospitalisation when necessary at times of crisis, helps build new confidence, strength and health within the patient and family. In this way a positive healthy reality can grow and emerge and not a world of fear or wish-fulfilment fantasy without foundation.

Where there are manic excitability problems, homoeopathy also helps, as long as there is some degree of cooperation and rapport from the patient. But where both remedy and physician seem part of a plot, conviction or conspiracy, then hospitalisation may be required under sedation until the patient regains sufficient basic trust to allay their suspicions (*Belladonna*, *Stramonium*, *Hyoscyamus*). Once the patient can accept the homoeopathic approach and work in an on-going way with the treating physician until stabilisation is reached, then there is every chance of a positive outcome.

Case Report

A man of 36 had been treated over several years for a recurrent schizophrenic problem. After several months of homoeopathic treatment he was apparently in total remission appearing perfectly rational and normal. The family suggested that he was well enough to discontinue treatment, but the patient confided that unknown to them, he had recently taken another overdose, after a minor row about smoking in the home. He was not suicidal at the time (*Aurum met*) and the overdose was clearly an expression of intense, yet suppressed feelings over family interference, which he was unable to cope with at the time. On the surface he was calm and unaggressive without the least expression of violence or rage (*Pulsatilla*). But with only minor provocation, his anger boiled over and turned dangerously into himself, resulting in inappropriate or self-destructive acts which could lead to tragedy. He had never fully been himself in any social situation because he lacked confidence (*Nat mur*). As a younger man he had been far too controlled and pseudo-mature (*Lycopodium*). All

64

of this contributed to the present problem. Homoeopathy was able to work with him at these levels and slowly help towards maturing the underlying causes. Fortunately he slept off the overdose, but it could easily have led to a fatality – as is common in this type of illness.

The patient obviously needed a further period of treatment and it was encouraging that he was able to tell me about the incident, discussing in some depth and insight why the episode had occurred. He needed homoeopathic support to tolerate and accept the inevitable differences of opinion and his ambivalent feelings, including anger to those close to him.

A woman aged eighty was treated for a severe irritating eczema. The reaction was probably triggered by contact with sprayed plants in her garden at a time of unusual family pressure, and when her husband was increasingly anxious and demanding. Homoeopathy helped her deal with the emotional issues more openly. Treatment took nearly two years for the skin to return to normal, because the reaction involved the whole of the body area, with swelling and a hide-like thickening of the skin causing intolerable irritation. Improvement occurred from top to bottom, in reverse order of development, so that the final area to cure and the slowest, was the original area of contact with the pesticide.

Allergy

Homoeopathy has an important and effective part to play in all allergic conditions, particularly hay-fever, migraine, allergic rhinitis and eczema. It can re-align an excessive or inappropriate physiological reaction at a protein sensitivity level as well as incorporating a balancing of psychological functioning. The single remedy, when well-chosen to fit the patient, can help to quickly resolve an often long-standing disability.

Common allergic problems involve food sensitivity to red meat (*Pyrogen*), milk (*Aethusa*), aluminium cooking utensils (*Alumina*), onions (*Thuja*), fat (*Pulsatilla*), coffee (*Causticum, Nux vomica, Ignatia*), tea (*Selenium*), beans and peas (*Bryonia*). Non-food allergens include pollen (the specific pollen in potency, e.g. *Timothy grass, Silver birch*), animal hair, house dust (*House dust*).

Where there is a problem which involves several generations of the family with perhaps asthma or eczema, then a miasm may be the underlying cause. Both Psora (*Sulphur*) and Sycosis (*Thuja*) are common in recurrent chronic skin or mucosal problems with irritation and thickening, or at other times, symptoms in the digestive and circulatory areas.

First-aid

Homoeopathy has proved invaluable over the years in the treatment of all the common first-aid emergencies that occur in the home. The remedy required naturally varies with the people and personalities involved, particularly in acute problems. In general, homoeopathy is remarkably effective in a wide variety of situations which vary from an insect sting, cut or graze to the treatment of infections, wounds, splinters, burns and scalds. In every case it is the degree of damage or trauma that decides whether homoeopathy is indicated as a treatment and judgement is required to match the remedy-profile to the symptoms with a minimum of delay. Severe cases may urgently require hospitalisation or treatment in a specialised unit, as with an extensive burn or severe road accident, with homoeopathy playing a less direct, more secondary role, to stimulate healing and a swifter return to recovery.

Casualty or Surgical Conditions

Where the problem is one which requires specialised care and treatment beyond the home and common first-aid approach then homoeopathy acts to support and strengthen vitality, minimising infection or reactions generally, other than the essential vital ones. In a surgical emergency, homoeopathy speeds cure by limiting shock or any adverse reaction to the initial accident, surgical intervention, loss of blood or fluids. It makes for a more responsive, confident and relaxed patient, with recovery-time kept to a minimum.

When there is an acute physical trauma or shock, loss of fluids are usually associated. These need to be urgently replaced intravenously without delay. *Arnica* or the Bach resuce remedy can be confidently given before hospitalisation and during the journey to a casualty department following a traffic or industrial injury. But homoeopathy is not magic, nor a panacea and it does not replace key conventional treatments when these are needed, better indicated or life-saving. Where there is an acute abdominal condition – appendicitis is a common example, then surgery is usually the treatment of choice and homoeopathy plays a secondary role to lessen shock (*Arnica*) bleeding (*Phosphorus*) and to support recovery from the tissue incision (*Staphisagria*).

Sometimes an operation is more of an elective procedure than an acute urgency, carried out on principles, or because it is policy, expedient, or a hygienic measure. Hysterectomy in a woman of 40 with fibroids may be recommended because she is out of the child-bearing age. In such cases homoeopathy may be an alternative to surgery as long as the menstrual loss is not excessive and a danger to life. For many, the decision whether to operate also depends upon feelings and wishes as well as the risk of illness. The patient often has profound feelings about her body, internal organs and a radical surgical approach. There are others who do not want to think or feel about such issues – they want to be guided by their doctor or the surgeon, and are happy to be advised and to totally hand over any decision to the specialists.

For the individual who does not want surgery, and where the physical problem is not urgent, or a danger to life, in many cases homoeopathy may help resolve the problem, or give a valuable breathing space, so that the patient has more time to watch how a problem is progressing. He can then decide what to do and which actions to take – under less pressure – based on his own wishes, feelings, instincts and knowledge.

But everyone is unique and the degree, severity,

rate of change of a physical condition, psychological balance and overall health are what eventually decides the best course of action. Where homoeopathy is tried before surgery – in a problem of tendon contracture (*Causticum*), cure often depends upon the causes and how long the condition has been present. The remedy used and the amount of vitality that can be stimulated or made available is also important. Results depend upon the quality of emotional resilience and the amount of stress present in the individual's life at the time.

Where an operation is felt to be mutilating or not strictly necessary, then homoeopathy can be usefully tried to see what changes are possible in the area affected as well as within the overall constitution and vitality.

For more chronic problems – diverticulitis, gall bladder disease, renal stones, low back syndrome, arthritis, rheumatism, spasm, indigestion, peptic ulcer or psoriasis, homoeopathy is often curative over a period of weeks or months – as long as there is not an obstructive basis to the condition or conventional methods more indicated.

Exhaustion States

In itself, homoeopathy cannot provide and replace depleted reserves. It can however bring about repose and essential relaxation so that a return to more healthy functioning occurs with replenishment of bodily reserves from food, the environment and a healthy atmosphere – providing that it is available. Both psychological as well as physical depletion occur with increasing frequency and

69

both need to be regularly replenished for life to continue at a high-level and to cope with demands. For such states, homoeopathy has a lot to offer and can make more energy available for the build-up of essential reserves. These are often the key to a return to health and more effective functioning in general.

Remedies to consider include – *China*, *Nux moschata*, *Opium*, *Kali carb*, *Arsenicum*, *Calcarea*, *Arnica*, *Phosphoric acid*.

Infection

These usually respond well to homoeopathy, particularly those of the bladder with cystitis, the chest in bronchitis, laryngitis, sore throat or asthma. Other common infective problems where there is a rapid response are skin problems – especially recurrent conditions – infected cuts and wounds, 'hang-nail' problems and sinusitis. In every case, provided that the infection falls within 'normal' or usual limits and is not one of overwhelming epidemic proportions, or involving an elderly person with diminished vitality, then the homoeopathic response is often favourable.

Pneumonia of the elderly, especially of an acute viral type is a difficult problem for any form of treatment. In general it is best treated by antibiotics with homoeopathy in a supportive, back-up role. Similarly, with major epidemics, or more unusual highly infectious conditions as cholera, typhoid, meningitis and smallpox – these are best treated in hospital with antibiotics, homoeopathy

70

reserved for background support and of most value in the convalescent phases of treatment.

Remedies which act on infection are *Hepar sulph*, *Merc sol*, *Pyrogen*, *Silicea*, *Belladonna*, *Lycopodium*, *Lachesis*. *Ant. crud* is another useful remedy for acute conditions, particularly of the skin. A nosode, such as *Tuberculinum* can be helpful in recurrent chest problems or *China* where there is an intermittent fever.

Deficiency Conditions

Homoeopathy can treat the milder deficiency diseases by giving the element or hormone lacking in homoeopathic potency. This is particularly valuable where there is sensitivity or intolerance of conventional and more gross forms of administration.

Common examples where homoeopathy is given as replacement therapy are:
Myxoedema (*Thyroidinum*)
Anaemia (*Ferrum met.*, *Folic ac*)
Vitamin Deficiency (the specific vitamin, eg Vitamin E in potency)
Hormonal imbalance (*Folliculinum*).

Pregnancy and Childbirth

Homoeopathy can help prevent early miscarriage where this is a recurrent problem and source of anxiety. During the latter half of pregnancy *Caulophyllum* is given in potency to stabilise the uterus, regularise contractions and to facilitate the

71

birth process. *Arnica* may also be given before and after the actual delivery to prevent excessive haemorrhage and shock.

During the Puerperium

After the delivery, it is not uncommon for the mother to experience a sense of flatness and let-down, varying in degree from a mild attack of the 'blues' to a full-blown puerperal psychosis. Homoeopathy is of value, whatever the level or intensity of the puerperal disturbance.

Sepia is of particular value at this time, especially where there are puzzling ambivalent feelings which become a source of guilt or confusion. When there has been a too rapid delivery or instruments were necessary for the delivery, with shock or bruising to the young infant, then *Arnica* is one of the best remedies, without risk for the baby.

Prevention

Homoeopathy has a major role to play in the prevention of epidemic disease where there has been a contact. It is of value in preventing the acute infections as German measles (*Rubella*), Whooping cough (*Pertussin*), Mumps (*Parotidinum*), Measles in the weak or convalescent child (*Morbillinum*), Shingles of the elderly, where a convalescent or weak adult has had contact with Chicken pox (*Varicellinum*) For the prevention of Scarlet Fever, *Belladonna* is the remedy of choice.

72

Chronic Problems

These are often recurrent problems that have failed to respond satisfactorily to a conventional approach and have become resistant to repeat prescriptions of perhaps steroids or antibiotics over the years. Problems include the chronic allergies – asthma, hay-fever, or the difficult 'civilisation' diseases like hiatus hernia, peptic-ulcer, raised blood pressure, colitis, angina. Homoeopathy is helpful in all of these unless surgery is required or the condition has been so left and neglected without treatment that the patient is in danger – as with the threat of a severe haemorrhage, or uncontrollable infection.

Case History

A patient was seen recently with a history of heart attacks and increasing severe anginal pain, occurring every hour of the day and night. The patient could not walk or speak without chest pain, and the least movement to undress or even describe the pain caused intolerable and severe chest pain. He was far too ill for a homoeopathic consultation and should have been in an acute cardiac unit several weeks previously, possibly on continuous anti-coagulant therapy.

It is unrealistic to expect homoeopathy to act as a miracle-cure – in a perilous condition which has been left to reach danger level and where the patient lacks the vitality and strength for a healing reaction to occur. It is always better to bring a patient for treatment as early as possible rather than to wait until the last possible moment or until he is in crisis.

CHAPTER SIX

The action and function of Homoeopathy

Homoeopathy acts at every age throughout life – from infancy to old age with a unique action, both physical and psychological. On the physical systems, it stimulates vital energy flow, elimination and mobilises reserves. On the psychological processes, it has a quite specific unlocking action, which leads to greater peace of mind and balance. This is best summarised by the following sections which explain in greater detail the unique and special properties of the homoeopathic prescription.

The Balancing function

Homoeopathy has an important role to play in correcting or balancing physiological functioning. Excesses of secretion and flow, whatever their cause, lead to problems, often with pain, spasm or colic and flatulence. All of these can be relieved or prevented by the homoeopathic approach which stimulates the body towards equilibrium, harmony and balance rather than passivity and stasis. Where an unsatisfactory state of intestinal or glandular inactivity prevails, indigestion or constipation are the inevitable outcome. The excessive build-up of either acidity, gas, tension, anger or resentment can be released as balancing occurs both psychologically as well as physiologically with increased relaxation and flow occurring at these levels. This lessening of emotional tension and anxiety leading to overall more centred perspectives is inseparable from the closely related glandular and intestinal functioning.

Homoeopathy matches the symptoms and variations of the individual, the major areas of physical and psychological activity at the time with the remedy profile. It harmonises with the individual and helps expose and correct immature or tense areas of limitation. A common example is where there has been an excessive attachment to a past trauma and hurt, or in some cases, a success, but inflated beyond significance to such an extent, that it blocks all further functioning and growth. The fear of a new hurt, or reluctance to leave past laurels, is often helped by *Natrum mur* or *Aconitum*, which act at this level.

Fixed attitudes and excessive attachments can pressurise the physical as well as psychological aspects of the person, so that challenging creative attitudes and imaginative perceptions are blocked or obstructed by rigidity. Physically, there may be a lessening of secretion and function, leading to problems of weakness, constipation, lack of drive, low levels of libido, pain, colic, acidity and flatulence. All may be helped by the homoeopathic approach which naturally brings the body towards equilibrium by it balancing action. Bottled-up tensions, anger or resentments are also released as the remedies help free spasm and blockage (*Nux vomica*). Lessening emotional tension and anxiety as well as physical tightness gives greater ease and relaxation generally, supporting more healthy glandular and intestinal functioning, reducing windy colic or flatulence.

Where there is failure of equilibrium and balance, physical or psychological negatives build up, leading to organic disease or a more definite emotional problem as phobia, depression, anxiety or loss of confidence. Because homoeopathy helps prevent the development and progression of unhealthy attitudes, it makes feeling and reactions easier to express and more spontaneous. In this way they cause less damage to the system, as the remedies help free self-expression and at the same time treat any associated physical condition.

The Strengthening function

Homoeopathy has a definite strengthening role to play which will consolidate and conserve energy so that it is more available where needed, supporting fitness and resistance, revitalising confidence and well-being. Increased vital energy is made available when and where it is needed. Patients feel better for homoeopathy, more relaxed and hopeful, as drive, bowel and sleep patterns improve and there is greater stamina and resistance at the same time as pain and tension lessen. This can be clearly

77

seen in a patient with a chronic back problem, weakness and pain. Often after a single prescription the patient may say 'look how much more I can do and how agile and strongly I can bend, move, or get out of a chair. I couldn't do that a week ago – my back was far too weak'. Psychologically it also strengthens confidence. *Arnica* is one of the best remedies to increase strength with *Arsenicum* a close second.

The Supportive Function

Homoeopathy supports the individual – as he or she is *now*, in the present, in expressions, growth, development, to expand and give out, to be more authentic as a person, more himself. It supports vital energies without provoking dissipation or depletion, mobilising essential energy for cure as far as it is inherently available in underfunctioning areas, stimulating circulation, physiological flow and release. It does not leave the patient exhausted, worse than before treatment or the original problem that brought him to the doctor in the first place. Supportive of each individual patient, it acts where most needed in the major areas of weakness and lack. It will not however act where there is not requirement of support or stimulus to functioning. A wrong inappropriate remedy usually has no untoward effect on the individual as a result, unless given repeatedly in very high potency.

Typical examples of supportive remedies are the use of *Caulophyllum* in pregnancy, *Sepia* for disturbed mother-infant relationships in either veterinary or human work, helping to balance ambivalent or negative feelings. *Ruta* acts on tendons and the supportive tissues of large joints, especially knee and hip. *Rhus tox* helps positively on the skin and articular contact areas of large and small joints. *Hepar sulph* supports healing throughout where there is an inflammatory reaction. *Symphytum* aids bone healing, as after a fracture. *Hypericum* is supportive to nervous tissue damage in general, especially the highly sensitive periosteal membrane surrounding the bone surfaces and vulnerable from a kick on the shin. *Arsenicum* counteracts weakness in general. More specifically, *Bryonia* acts strongly on respiratory functioning. *Arnica* supports swollen, painful and bruised areas of soft tissue damage where there has been bleeding. *Ignatia* relieves the acute psychological pain of separation, grief and loss. None of the remedies cause suppression of a problem or limit awareness of feelings involved.

Preservative function

Homoeopathy acts to preserve and support greater integration and togetherness of the patient with positive strengthening of identity, aims, drive, self-confidence and the will to get well. It helps preserve and store drive and vitality physically as well as psychologically so that these can be built-up and added to. In this way both the physical and psychological integrity of the person is preserved for the reconstruction of better health and a more authentic individuality.

Homoeopathy has the power to mobilise, concentrate and redistribute whatever vitality the individual has at their disposal and directs their energies to the areas most needed.

Homoeopathy has the potential to unlock and bring into the open half-formed, sometimes chronic or repetitive symptoms which recur as odd or brief illnesses, often with no clear-cut clinical identity or tangible meaning. Such vague problems, may seem to occur in apparent isolation or to engender nausea, exhaustion, indigestion, constipation, insomnia or fainting. The homoeopathic approach brings them out more so that they can be better treated and integrated into the patient totality, in this way less isolated and more part of overall treatment. The re-emergence of suppressed symptoms helps the patient and also the prescriber to be more accurate in choice of a subsequent remedy and depth of potency.

Un-locking function

All too often problems get locked-away in minor areas of the body which like motor-way slipways cannot be reached so that a chronic situation develops. In fact, the problem lies just beneath the surface, but inaccessible to natural healing responses which are unable to function there. The problem is contained, but cannot be released. This is seen particularly whenever there has been a prolonged treatment by one of the steroid drugs. The disease is kept alive but immobilised, partially paralysed, under the body's defensive layer – as can be clearly seen in many cases of chronic eczema or psoriasis. The condition neither evolves and cures nor clears-up, apparently stable as long as the tablets and creams are continued. However if these are missed for more than a few days, then the whole problem breaks through the surface with a vengeance and irritating severity, only to be pushed back and down again with a different suppressant or higher dose of the original drug.

This tendency for diseases to 'have out', or to come out and express themselves is a perfectly natural vital reaction. After stopping suppressant therapy, such emergent reactions may be more severe and are sometimes a source of considerable anxiety to the patient. With homoeopathy chronic patterns and processes become unlocked and made available to the natural healing powers of the body – which the remedy stimulates. But when there is a long history of suppression from whatever cause, then the initial healing reaction is likely in all cases to be a strong one until the state of harmony and balance is re-established.

A recurrent problem, either physical or emotional, is usually the result of past suppression, blockage or denial. Homoeopathy helps break down the barriers which immure and isolate such fragments of disease, integrating them into a more meaningful, less isolated totality, which makes it more amenable to cure.

In cancer, the body attempts to encapsulate and isolate an abnormal galloping cellular division process, so that it can be kept within boundaries – sometimes by processes of calcification or ossification, where the growth is slow growing. For stoney-hard conditions, *Bryonia* is often the treatment of choice, the remedy supporting overall healing and balance for hard lumps, especially of the breast. In some tumours, this walling-up of a pathological condition is totally successful. It also occurs in cases where there is a chronic abscess condition – tuberculosis, or certain parasitic cystic conditions. It sometimes happens that the centre of these encapsulated areas, although largely starved of circulation and vitality, is still dormant and a cause of obscure toxic problems of varying degrees of intensity. For such cases homoeopathy helps drain and break down the area, so that it can be more thoroughly and permanently treated by homoeopathy or other methods, including anti-biotics when necessary, so that a thorough cure is finally established. Major unlocking remedies include *Sulphur*, *Silicea*, *Tuberculinum* and the nosodes, but they need to be used with care and caution and preferably only by a physician.

Where an old TB condition has been dormant and immured within a cyst or scar area over the years, homoeopathy may provoke its re-emergence, as the capsule is broken-down. Depending upon the age and vitality of the patient, It may or may not be a positive desirable step to take. This is why very careful clinical judgement and experience are needed when prescribing homoeopathy when there is a history of such conditions. In a similar way, with a barely con-tained emotional storm or psychological illness, this could also be opened up again by the potencies and lead to a reaction. Clinical judgement is needed in all of these problems and illustrates the importance of taking a full past history of disease and family health in every case. It is essential to carefully appraise whether it is in a patients best interest for a dormant condition to be released and whether the individual should be re-exposed to the risks of a past condition when reserves of health and balance are uncertain. If there is doubt, then the use of high potency unlocking remedies for such problems is contra-indicated and best avoided until the patient can be more carefully monitored, or reserves built-up and available again.

Curative Function

By unlocking and bringing to the surface, both mental and physical spheres, homoeopathy makes every disease process more accessible to the inherent natural processes of cure, within the individual. Homoeopathy can give rapid relief to many acute and painful physical conditions, as colic, toothache, neuralgia, otitis media, tonsillitis, cystitis, abscess, boil, lumbago, depending upon degree and severity – often within a few hours. At times relief comes within minutes of taking the remedy depending upon individual sensitivity to the homoeopathic stimulus. It can also relieve chronic, more long-standing problems of indigestion, angina, hypertension (blood pressure), provided that the remedy chosen is one which works at both the source and origin of the problem as well as on the prevailing symptoms.

A change of priorities, aims and drives may be necessary when these are unhealthy or undermining, contributing to an illness process. Accident-proness (*Kali carb*), recurrent sprains (*Calcarea*), pain or spasm from a sports injury (*Arnica, Nux vomica, Ruta*) are often associated with self-defeating damaging attitudes, pushing the individual too much to win or to be best always, but undermining joy, ease, pleasure and relaxation.

Because homoeopathy respects the needs of the individual, it will not normally liberate a negative process, unless this is in the interests of the whole person, and can be dealt with adequately by the body's defences at the time. The homoeopathic stimulus acts through the defensive immune system, mobilising it to activity. But where this channel is immobilised by the steroid group of drugs or by an immune-deficiency disease (AIDS), its effects are undermined or neutralised and it is less effective.

Centreing Function

This is an important major area of activity of the homoeopathic remedies that is not always appreciated. Centreing the patient allows more overall less distorted viewpoints to be taken, helping ease and relaxation, but keeping priority of need to the fore. Each remedy has the ability to centre psychologically as well as physically because of the inherent action of the potencies within the mental sphere as well as the physical. This is most marked when the higher potencies are used.

In this way, the patient is less likely to be overwhelmed by trivial insignificant pressures and energy can be more positively directed. Every homoeopathic remedy works to lessen or limit an extreme position – the physical tension and hardness of an acute boil, or taking the steam out of an over-intense emotional reaction, making for a more balanced overall position, optimum for cure.

Case Reports

A woman came with a double problem – she had a strangulated haemorrhoid or 'pile', the size and appearance of a ripe victoria plum, painful in the extreme and making sitting impossible, walking difficult. But she was also severely depressed – quite unrelated to her painful rectal condition. Within a few hours of receiving *Pulsatilla* in the IOM potency, the pile had shrunk to a small size and became more comfortable and bearable. At the same time confidence returned following a long talk with her boy-friend about a matter that had been troubling her and causing conflict for several weeks. This latter problem had been both worrying and depressing her and had threatened to undermine her basic confidence. She was able to suddenly feel herself for the first time in months, to resolve the psychological situation and regain confidence so that almost immediately she felt better, more of a person and in balance. The condition was resolved in both areas by the single treatment and no further help or other remedies were required.

Another patient came with a severe anxiety-tension state, unable to sleep or to relax. At the same time there was the most severe urinary problem of intense irritation with an intense cystitis causing painful frequency of urination every 15 minutes, both day and night. A single dose of *Sycotico 30* was given – one of the bowel nosodes.

Within minutes, the patient experienced relief for the first time in weeks, the psychological state more relaxed at the same time as the bladder condition. My patient fell into a deep refreshing sleep after taking the remedy and both bladder and tension state completely cleared from that time with no repeat of remedy required.

The Dynamic function of cure

The law of cure is well-known and clearly seen throughout homoeopathic treatments. It is often more noticeable in skin and arthritic conditions or where there is a rheumatic problem. Most recent symptoms respond first to treatment and those problems that have been present for long periods respond only later to the potencies – the remedy going 'back in time' so to speak, rooting-out step by step the deepest and initial causes of an illness. Homoeopathy often brings to the surface during cure, old long-forgotten symptoms that just as rapidly, disappear as quickly as they arise – either spontaneously or with the helping hand of a new remedy. The recurrence of these symptoms does not mean that the patient is getting worse or having a recurrence of an old problem, but it does mean that the remedy is acting dynamically and deeply on the remnants of earlier conditions – not dealt with adequately at that time, or perhaps suppressed. These can now be finally eradicated from the body's vital resources, bringing back a welcome boost to vitality which was otherwise being sapped and drained-away. Once out in the 'open', such symptoms are quite naturally erased by nature's healing resources.

Symptoms are also normally relieved from the top of the body downwards – from scalp to trunk and finally the feet in keeping with the direction of energy flows. Recovery also occurs from more centrally affected organs as the heart, kidney, liver or lungs to more peripheral and relatively insignificant areas as a joint-capsule or muscle. This is not always clear to the patient. A heart condition such as angina may clear up, but the patient says he is no better or feels even worse because he had developed a recurrence of an old indigestion problem or a frozen shoulder. But the heart is healthier, and the patient free from pain on walking.

The process of homoeopathy is such that it will unerringly flush-out any disease process in its path at the particular depth and resonance of the remedy and potency used, according to the physiology of the areas being cleared and re-vitalised.

Some further general points about the action of the remedies

Note that the specific action of every homoeopathic remedy is to 'throw out' all that is repressed or suppressed, beneath the surface and unavailable to the patient at either a physical or psychological level. The remedy brings these physical symptoms to the surface, making them 'available' to the body for resolution and cure. The remedy does not however differentiate between

87

the elements that it liberates, either good, positive and desirable or what may be undesirable or painful. At times a remedy may throw-out past feelings of grievance, anger and resentment, deep forgotten memories or feelings of need, which may have blocked creative drives. This is all part of the uniqueness of the homoeopathic response and why it is particularly important to follow-up the initial prescription closely and carefully, especially a high-potency one. The patient may need guidance with their psychological reactions – positive or negative which emerge. Caution is only necessary, as in all medical treatments or healing, where there is a previous history of severe or chronic disease, particularly a poorly resolved and immured old T.B. condition, a previous psychiatric history of breakdown, or cancer.

CHAPTER SEVEN

Dilution and disease

Homoeopathy operates according to profound physiological principles existing throughout nature in both animal and human life. These principles are clearly expressed by the Schultz law of stimulus and growth which states that where there are healthy living growing cells, these are stimulated by a small stimulus, inhibited by a medium one and that a strong stimulus destroys all life and growth. Much of this work was carried out by the experimental physiologists Arndt and Schultz, working with yeast cells and the effect of arsenic on their proliferation. Arsenic as *Arsenicum* in its homoeopathic form, is also a very deep-acting powerful remedy, one used extensively in acute conditions. There is no doubt about the importance of this principle.

The trace elements are essential to healthy functioning, and the body, which can synthesise most things is unable to produce its own trace-substances as copper and cadmium. These are needed in minute amounts for the formation of blood and other cell-tissues. Without them, the body becomes prone to diseases. It is also well-known that both copper and cadmium are extremely toxic in large doses to the body, but in their minute stimulating 'homoeopathic' dietary amounts, they are absolutely essential to health.

Homoeopathic remedies are always given in small dosages because these can be most easily responded to and taken-up by the body. They are used by the body as 'pointers' to tension or lack, directing vitality to the areas of most need, opening-up any illness areas to the body's intrinsic healing powers. Where there is a mineral or vitamin deficiency, the substance in its homoeopathic form can be taken-up and absorbed by the body without excessive loss of the substance in the stool or causing intolerable irritation to the sensitive lining mucosa of the stomach or bowel.

Homoeopathy acts by the principle of using a minimal dilution, repeated as infrequently as possible. The aim in homoeopathy is only one – to stimulate a healing response in the area affected so that a break through of energy-activity can occur and then to stop the remedy as soon as possible.

Originally they were given in their mother-tincture undiluted form by Hahnemann and his followers, which, although provoking a powerful vital reaction, had undesirable side-effects too from the strength of the tinctures used. He began experimenting with weaker solutions, increasing the serial dilutions, to find one that would be effective without side-effects. To the amazement of Hahnemann the remedies were enhanced in their action by serial dilution. The more he 'stretched' or diluted the potency – rather than weakening the homoeopathic action – like an elastic band, its power was increased. This chance finding, seemingly paradoxical at the time, led to a new dimension of thinking and homoeopathic development for both patient and doctor.

By bringing vitality, healing, circulation and warmth to parts previously inert or non-active, the remedies transform areas of disease into healthy tissue again. A non-functioning part, with loss of tone or spasm, pain and blockage, may become vital tissue again within a short period of time. Once the healing reaction has occurred, the homoeopath has done his work, restoring vitality where previously there was tension which the body could neither eliminate nor contain without symptom-formation or interference with normal functioning. The stimulated vital reaction can in most cases be relied upon to continue and carry-on to complete the work. Homoeopathy acts like a key – opening a door and pointing the way in areas where previously there was no way-apparent, no lock or even key-hole visible in what seemed an impossible situation. This is why patients are so often completely astounded by their speed of response to the remedies, particularly when the higher potencies (centesimal) are given.

The lower dilutions (decimal) (3x or 6c) act at a more tangible physical and tissue levels with any general constitutional action secondary to local peripheral ones.

When the higher dilutions (30c and more) are prescribed, there is more stimulus of general activity, with responses at both the mental and physical levels. Where a problem is apparently at shoulder level only, due to penetration of cold or damp into the joint, then *Sanguinaria*, *Rhus tox*, or *Dulcamara*, according to the symptoms, in their lower, 'local' potencies is a perfectly adequate treatment. But when the problem is a 'frozen' shoulder with clear psychological undertones – following the loss of a close relative or from an unhappy marriage, with barely controlled anger, rage and resentment, then the prescription has to be considered more deeply. In cases where such underlying emotions are present at the expense of health, the higher 30 even 200c potencies give better results and enable an underlying depression to be resolved more speedily.

Minimal doses of dilution are becoming increasingly important in other wider fields than those of medicine. In agriculture and the prevention of toxic damage to plants and animals it has become increasingly recognized as a major area of research and disease-prevention. A recent paper (1979) in the Annals of Human Biology describes the importance of garlic in plant health as an effective fungicide and pesticide at dilutions of one part in a hundred – which is the beginning of our centesimal scale in homoeopathy. In Smarden (Kent), an outbreak of poisoning occurred in the early 60's when many cattle had to be slaughtered and burned. There was a small leak from a nearby manufacturing company into a stream which also fed an animal water-supply. Fluoracetamide was being manufactured and a dilution of one part in 10 million or 10^{-7} was lethal. This level of dilution is equivalent to the higher potencies used in homoeopathy and confirms directly that such dilutions not only act as a stimulus to healing, but in certain cases – as with the fluoracetamide, they can be lethal too.

Such dangers are fortunately not the case in homoeopathy where standards of purity and safety are of the highest. Stringent safeguards are in operation to ensure total non-toxicity. This is why there are no known side-effects of the method or from the remedies used. Safety is assured at all ages and in all dosages.

CHAPTER EIGHT

The advantages of the homoeopathic approach

Homoeopathy uses fundamental light energy of solar origin, inherent within the mother substance to achieve its therapeutic functioning. This energy is mobilised and made available for the patient by successive serial dilutions and succussion (vigorous shaking) of the potency at each stage of preparation. This primary energy acts as a trigger to stimulate individual energy flows. The minute amount of ultimate energy substance resonates with areas of growth and flow blockage according to the identity or configuration of the remedy chosen. Such changes are made possible because of the homoeopathic pharmacist's unique way of preparing the remedies, imprinting upon them the molecular configuration or energy potential of the mother substance. In this way the remedies differ considerably from a simple tincture or herbal solution, being far more dynamic and active, rapidly absorbed and acceptable to the body's vital system with a richer deeper therapeutic potential.

Homoeopathy is a natural method using natural substances and principles, in tune with the biological functioning of the individual, capable of acting at cellular and psychological levels within the patient. It also differs from most allopathic or synthetic drugs, which are essentially non-biological in action, chemical in origin and never really in resonance with the body as a totality. Many of our most advanced and modern treatments give unpredictable results, stimulating a temporary often shifting 'synthetic' cure because they are out of phase with the needs and total expressions of the patient.

Homoeopathy is in resonance with the overall personality, the total man and treatment like the cure, forms part of a meaningful unity.

To some degree, everyone has natural vital resources within them which support change and healing. These are generally bound within the constitutional profile and body reserves, but made more available by the remedy, which acts as a catalyst towards balance and cure. This inherent homoeopathic releasing function often points the direction of treatment to be initiated – loosening any knots created by the individual psychology, or from social and family pressures as well as the pulls of genetic inheritence.

Homoeopathy stimulates the resources of the body to bring about a cure in its own time, by its own rhythms, without imposing a pattern of responses which the individual is unable to cope with, or respond to. Each patient proceeds according to his own vital energy resources and reserves. Some establish a rapid and energetic vital response, others respond more slowly and gently in keeping with their speed of overall psychological and physiological reactions. In homoeopathy, no standards or pressures are laid down, the body is simply stimulated along certain predictable pathways of response and allowed to proceed at its own pace. This is why the question 'How long will it take doctor'? is difficult to answer unless there is already experience of the patient, knowledge of his responses – perhaps of a particular remedy or constitutional prescription. When the patient is in a convalescent state, the remedies still work, but more time is needed and a slower response is the norm and to be expected.

Because homoeopathy is not an exhausting treatment draining vitality and reserves it does not provide extra work for the vital kidneys and liver organs as it stimulates evacuation, neutralisation and detoxification. Homoeopathy preserves energy flows without side-effects and is why it is effective at all ages from the child of a few weeks old to the most senior elder of the family.

The whooping cough prophylactic nosode *Pertussin* is usually active in the youngest infant. Equally the prostatic remedy *Sabal serr*, is effective in the ocotogenerian or when an elderly lady has a touch of bladder weakness with a tendency to 'leak' slightly when rushing or coughing. Whatever the age, the well-chosen remedy will always strengthen and act to some degree, however much the calendar has turned. Every age is seen in the busy practice, often several generations of the same family, each with a characteristic problem common to their particular age-group. I often see whole families in consultation, grandparents, mums and dads and children – all responding individually, with the single remedy just as effective in the elderly as in the baby.

Remedies stimulate a general state of well-being and of confidence generally without leaving the patient more depleted and in a worse state than before, worse than the original condition being treated – as can frequently happen with some vaccination reactions in the young child.

The remedies are pleasant to take, usually made-up in sucrose pills or granules and quite acceptable to the youngest infant or most difficult child. Once swallowed they do not lead to a foul taste or breath, a coated tongue or any after-taste or after-effects other than the intended ones.

There are no side-effects from the remedies, as diarrhoea, nausea, weakness, circulatory effects, haemorrhagic tendencies, drowsiness which could be either overwhelming or dangerous. Frequently it stimulates a temporary aggravation of an underlying problem – as part of the reaction which the homoeopath is aiming for. This may give discomfort before an improvement occurs. However such vital responses are different from a side-reaction to a synthetic drug treatment where there is intolerance or allergy to the remedy. This does not occur in homoeopathy and the aggravations felt are easily understood by the patient as positive and part of cure.

There is no danger from homoeopathy because the degree of dilution is aimed at giving the patient an infinitesimal stimulus. Because the aim is always the smallest effective dose, this is also a safe one with a minimum of external outside interference upon the body which, creates and emphasises a maximum of 'self' or natural cure and confidence.

A remedy does not have to be taken for tedious endless periods with a maintainance dosage to sap energy or promote psychological dependency, which undermines health over years. As soon as there is a recovery and a return to normal function- ing, whatever the problem, the remedy is stopped and the body's natural functioning encouraged to resume as before.

The remedies can be used preventatively or prophylacticaly in certain problems. For example, German measles of pregnancy, Scarlet fever, Whooping cough, Measles or when the individual is in an especially low vulnerable state or a particu- lar disease is epidemic at the time. It is also useful when there is a potential danger to health as with Influenza of the elderly or a young infant.

Homoeopathy acts deeply and will eradicate the roots of a disease, even when chronic, present since birth or with a family-tendency to the condition. Especially it has the ability to 'sweep out' cleanly and deeply within the tissues, remnants of earlier inadequately treated or suppressed problems. At the time they seemed cured but nevertheless have recurred in one form or other over the years as a constant irritant lowering vitality and health. This 'cleaning-out' role of homoeopathy may bring to the surface elements of a former illness. A condi- tion, long forgotten, may 'hang around' over the years, not unlike a skeleton in the cupboard, a recurrent problem only finally eradicated and cured by the new found vitality of the appropriate remedy.

In chronic disease or where there is an inherited tendency to weakness, homoeopathy offers a radical cure for many conditions, though the symptoms may not always form a tangible clinical entity.

Increasingly the busy practitioner sees an ever-growing number of chronic or recurrent problems in the surgery. Recent (1985) figures show a higher incidence in the U.K. than in other areas of the European community for male circulatory and heart disease, accounting for 54% of all mortality. In one form or other, these are by far the commonest problems seen, especially blood-pressure, coronary thrombosis, sluggish circulation, palpitations, angina or irregular heart beat. Such problems are always aggravated by obesity, smoking, a high-fat diet and lack of exercise. Not uncommonly liver, lung or kidney complications are associated.

A family history of heart disease, means that even greater attention should be given to illness prevention, especially by weight correction and regular exercise. Other chronic conditions seen, but not directly circulatory, are peptic ulceration, indigestion, constipation, diverticulitis, colitis, diabetes, gall-bladder disease, hernia, arthritis or rheumatism, chronic sinus problems, asthma, bronchitis and emphysema. Allergic diseases of every type are the other group of chronic illnesses seen daily.

Many respond to simple reassurance and more information about diet, exercise, a reduction in cigarette and alcohol intake. For others, the problems are more deeply entrenched, becoming worse when conventional remedies are taken. They may not respond to homoeopathy, because it was prescribed too late during the progress of a disease or reserves were too depleted for a satisfactory response, the patient already exhaused at the start of therapy.

The problem of chronic illness is often that the origins are not clear or if known, not acknowledged and perceived by the patient. Often too many years have elapsed since the disease process started and multiple treatments have – like the illness process – eroded health. This leads inevitably to a gradual pathway of decline. Because the origins are not admitted, wrong information is given to the doctor, and what is elicited from the patient is too descriptive or superficial. Levels of communication and interchange in the surgery tend to be at a trivial level from pressure of time or fear of appearing foolish. The dialogue between doctor and patient is too often at a purely factual level only – about how the tablets are affecting him – rather than the true and relevant contributory causes.

One reason why the homoeopathic consultation is so detailed and time-consuming, is the importance of going back to fundamentals and origins with every patient. This is basic if there is going to be any chance of a chronic condition being resolved and prescribed for in a way that gives lasting results.

Insight into the true reasons for a chronic problem is too often lacking and doctor, family, and patient may collude for months, even years to avoid looking at the real roots of a problem which are felt to be too embarrassing or painful. But behind every chronic problem a reason exists and there must be awareness of this somewhere within the patient's grasp, if memory or insight can be stimulated or permitted. Homoeopathy aims to facilitate just such understanding and a return to basics by a series of related prescriptions which take the patient back through successive layers. As these are freed, they are made available for awareness and treatment.

The management of a chronic problem is never an easy one because it is long-standing with vitality usually reduced by ineffective treatments over the years. These have often undermined confidence and drive over the years, depending upon degree and causes. Homoeopathy offers an approach which can radically change the position, leading to a gradual easing of symptoms and a cure. Where the origins and causes are known, these can be immediately treated by the remedies, even where the original damage goes back many years. The homoeopathic potency acts to loosen-up and to free the patient in their major areas of non-functioning which led to the build-up of a problem. Causative factors from the past include fear (*Aconitum*), grief and loss (*Ignatia*), viral infections and Influenza (*Influenzinum*), injury with perhaps a fall or shock (*Arnica*), head injury or concussion (*Helleborus*), post-vaccination reactions (*Thuja*).

In this way, homoeopathy acts in depth and at a causative level within the constitutional make-up of the patient and where it most accurately fits the particular individual. A positive reaction of health occurs in areas where previously there was only depressing limitation, repetition, depletion and non-function. Homoeopathy helps heal the gulf

101

between a diseased area of the body and any dis-ease of functioning as an effective person, because it stimulates integration of both into a more healthy whole.

With chronic illness problems, remedies are usually given over several months, based on the clinical picture at the time, using a variety of potencies according to symptoms and the degree of response or reaction evoked.

The individual constitutional remedy, with its powerful ability to restore a harmonising totality is of particular value in chronic disease and is almost certainly needed at some point in treatment.

CHAPTER NINE

Some limitations too

In reality these are relatively few and mainly centred around problems which are obstructive or surgical in origin, or where the intrinsic individual vitality, for whatever reason, is abnormally weak or unavailable.

1. The method is not recommended for a primarily surgical condition as acute appendicitis, or where there is severe abdominal infection with the risk of peritonitis occurring. Where an acute severe haemorrhage has occurred or an imminent danger, or for any condition whatsoever which requires surgery, homoeopathy should be in a supportive role only. Homoeopathy acts as a gentle stimulus to the body's healing powers. Where an acute condition has arisen, for whatever reason and is overwhelming, entering deeply into organs or eroding tissues, then usually the homoeopathic approach has been left too late and immediate surgical or antibiotic treatment should be used to help the patient. In such situations, homoeopathic remedies play a secondary and background role to conventional methods. The underlying reason as to

why the tissues have become weak or non-vital can be left to a later post-convalescent time and then dealt with by the homoeopathic approach.

2. When there is an acute illness crisis as with an overwhelming infection, the body not responding in a healthy way with a temperature or inflammatory reaction, or the patient is toxic, weak or elderly, lacking in reserves, then a homoeopathic approach should be used with caution. Conventional treatments are usually indicated in the initial stages.

3. In general, whenever the usual defensive reactions of the body fail to contain, limit or localise an infection, then homoeopathy is not usually the ideal treatment at this stage. A period of time is needed to build-up energy reserves which may take several weeks. During this period of build-up, the patient may be dangerously vulnerable and homoeopathy is best left until the crisis is well and truly over.

4. Homoeopathy is not a panacea or a cure-all. Anyone who pretends it is does not understand the method fundamentally and does the treatment a disservice. It is important that the indications to prescribe are clear-cut and take into account the patient's ability to respond to the remedies and the length of time that this is likely to take.

The tablets should not be handled because the medicine is on the surface and this lessens their efficacy or may neutralise them completely. They are best avoided during a period of steroid treatment or immediately after it. An excessive intake of tea or coffee also reduces the homoeopathic action. It is not recommended to take any form of suppressant treatment at the same time as a homoeopathic one because they neutralise and have an opposite effect upon the remedies. Treatment is often best delayed until they have been stopped.

CHAPTER TEN

More indications for homoeopathy

Homoeopathy is perhaps most active in the group of illnesses, aptly called the diseases of civilisation. These form a rather untidy *pot pourri* of maladaptions, depleted drives and physiological mal organisations, frequently the result of a faulty diet or unnatural life-style. Because of multiple often damaging treatments over the years, from lack of exercise and the side-effects of the social stimulants – coffee, tea, alcohol and tobacco, the whole organism is in a stagnant state of physiological functioning. Obesity is commonly the result of an inharmonious life-style and a major contributing factor to the problem. In general there is a faulty adjustment to the demands and needs of modern living with alienation from deeper concerns and the spiritual. This gives the essential balance needed to remain healthy in a largely concrete and externally functioning insensitive society.

Often these civilisation illnesses cannot be given a clear-cut clinical nomenclature or diagnosis because they are so vague, varied, and fragmentary in nature. Included are the common problems of constipation, exhaustion, indigestion, nausea, lack of drive, energy and libido, depression, poor circulation, rheumatism, premature aging, and many uterine and prostate difficulties.

Homoeopathy is clearly not indicated for tuberculosis, syphilis, typhoid, cholera, meningitis or any of the highly infectious epidemic conditions, including parasitic disease, where there is a safe effective modern alternative available which does not put the patient more at risk than the disease itself as a result of treatment.

In general, homoeopathy is most indicated for conditions where physically or psychologically, over a period of weeks or months, there has been a build-up of stress and tension. To be effective, the underlying problem should not be one which is either completely mechanical or surgical in origin, nor related to an acute or overwhelming infection.

Invasive tumours and cancers are conditions where natural immunity and resistance to abnormal cellular division has been lost. They are often associated with long-standing negative attitudes linked to self-neglect or a suppression of personal feelings. Homoeopathy may be indicated for cancer in a supportive general way or at times in a more defined specific role according to the needs of the individual patient, the extent and rapidity of spread of the disease. It can play a complementary role, working in tandem with modern medical techniques which involve the use of cytotoxic drugs or more classical, metaphysical approaches as visualisation which are also effective. Homoeopathy supports and maximises such contrasting therapies where a global approach is needed for the patient. Mistletoe in potency as *Ischador* M or Q, has given good results over the years in these conditions – taken orally or locally injected into the area affected.

Diet, counselling, acupuncture, meditation and relaxation treatments as well as opiates may also be needed. These may help to treat pain, put the patient into an optimum position for cure and give the homoeopathic potency the best possible chance to stimulate a curative reaction.

The best approach to cancer is undoubtedly prevention and every year progress is made in this field with new specific tests developed and evolved. The cervical smear test is undoubtedly the best example of progress in an area where cancer is notoriously difficult to diagnose and treat early, because symptoms are often only produced at a late stage. Body scan, ultrasound and new x-ray techniques are being evolved in a similar way using the principles of detecting early cellular changes and mutations from saliva, urine and gastic mucosa. These will eventually also provide a screening profile as effective and simple as the smear test. All of these are important because they detect changes within cells before symptoms of the disease develop at a pre-cancer stage. This allows relatively simple treatments, such as Laser techniques at the earliest stages.

The homoeopathic patient should not neglect such advances or regular clinical check-ups. A thorough breast self-examination and palpation is recommended every three months for every woman in order to detect any lumps which may occur – whatever their cause. This preventative approach should work in harmony with the homoeopathic one and treatment. Homoeopathy should complement modern medical techniques and not try to compete or be an alternative to them.

Homoeopathy is indicated as long as the patient is not too weak, with too little vitality to respond to the powerful stimulus that each remedy gives. When a condition is terminal, homoeopathy can help smooth the way, giving the patient dignity to the end, reducing the amount of pain-relieving drugs and avoiding confusion or numbing of senses and awareness. The high potencies are generally best avoided in terminal care patients and a 6c or 30c dilution gives serenity with clarity of mind. Only in the very early stages is it wise to give the higher potencies and these should always be at the discretion of the homoeopathic doctor.

In young people, prevention of disease should be emphasised by highlighting the dangers of a stressful life-style. At all ages, diet should be both nutritious and balanced. Where there is a family history of cancer or heart disease, then exposure to such irritants as tobacco smoke or alcohol in excess should be minimal. The risks of hormonal imbalance as a result of the contraceptive pill should also be carefully considered. These are often better replaced by a more straightforward barrier method from time to time.

The family as a whole should try to discuss how their overall state of health can be further improved and any reasons why a chronic problem is perpetuated. They should also explore why social props and addictions are necessary and how these can be best reduced or avoided.

Homoeopathy is not an alternative to conventional medicine and surgery when required and they should never be delayed because of it. When applied with skill and experience, conventional medicine is life saving and essential. Where homoeopathy is clearly not indicated as the first treatment of choice, it can nevertheless support and maximise the action of a vital conventional treatment, as long as it is not a suppressant. Where a conventional approach is not working well or has failed, then an alternative approach, such as homoeopathy, may be the principle treatment of choice. Sometimes it is necessary to combine homoeopathy with conventional treatments as well as other holistic ones. Whenever possible the homoeopathic potencies should be taken at a different time from conventional remedies and also stored separately from them.

In every case, the supportive homoeopathic approach puts the patient more at ease, more relaxed and comfortable, lessening tension and suffering, as well as giving a better outlook which is fundamental to every cure.

First-aid conditions respond well provided they are not severe and extensive with a major laceration. A severe burn, scald, wound or haemorrhage that requires suturing should have hospital treatment, but others respond well to the homoeopathic approach. If an ambulance is necessary, homoeopathy supports the patient before it arrives, reducing shock and helping to prevent complications. Homoeopathy will also reduce infection and haemorrhage. But in every first-aid case it is important to be realistic and to use judgement as to the extent of the injury and whether or not it is suitable for homoeopathy. When there is doubt, or no immediate response to the remedies, get another opinion from the nearest casualty department without loss of time.

Homoeopathy is used effectively for menstrual disorders, problems of heart and circulation including blood-pressure, digestive difficulties and urinary problems. Muscular cramps, rheumatism and arthritis also respond well and are frequently relieved or cured. Other important areas of reaction are infection of the skin, nose, throat and chest. Many common skin conditions such as acne and psoriasis also clear completely with homoeopathy.

Emotional conditions – tension and anguish are among the foremost indications for homoeopathy, especially where diminished vitality and a build-up of fatigue, exhaustion and apathy have occurred. Such stress conditions diminish resistance and the body's natural immune-defences.

Where vitality reserves are low, homoeopathy correctly applied, can work wonders to pull the person round from a vulnerable position. When recovery seems prolonged, even impossible to attain after a severe infection which has 'emptied the batteries' it is particularly valuable, although slower in action.

Circulatory and catarrhal conditions respond well and peptic ulceration is frequently helped, provided that the condition is not one that has been neglected to the point of perforation, or

111

where scar tissue has formed an obstruction which only surgery can put right. Such complications although rare, must be ruled out at the time of consultation and examination. Where there is doubt, a barium meal or other radiological investigation may be essential. Duodenitis, duodenal ulceration, hiatus hernia, gall-bladder dysfunction respond positively, but where gall-bladder symptoms are due to a large stone causing obstruction, colic and an impaired flow of bile along its duct, then surgery is recommended with homoeopathy in a back-up role.

All the stress diseases respond well to homoeopathy. These are unfortunately now as common in our domestic pets as in humans, which is one of the reasons why veterinary homoeopathy has become so popular. The very clear-cut response from animals of all kinds scuttles criticism of the method, based on ignorance and misinformation, which suggests that homoeopathy is suggestion or a placebo-response with no true healing by the remedies.

Eczema, psoriasis, chronic skin infective conditions and fungal states, respond well to homoeopathy, sometimes after an aggravation where suppressants have been used. Herpes – as shingles (herpes zoster), or its genital form, is becoming increasingly a matter of concern, especially the latter, in many young people. Many carriers are symptom-free. Both are largely incurable by conventional methods but can respond positively to homoeopathy. The other form of herpes is more benign although unpleasant – I refer to oral herpes or 'cold sore' of the lips and mouth. Position and site indicate the specific homoeopathic treatment required.

Many intimate difficulties within the couple's relationship and sexual sphere respond well to a homoeopathic approach when combined with adequate time to explore the problem. Often the couple are best seen jointly. Problems include lack of interest – sometimes associated with the contraceptive 'pill', pain, spasm, frigidity, premature ejaculation and impotency. All may be helped by the remedies because the potencies act in the sexual sphere and help mature immature attitudes and distortions. There is often a basic lack of communication at this level because of shame, guilt, confusion, shyness or lack of information which needs to be overcome.

Because of the depth and action of the remedy in the psychological sphere, it gives many unique advantages. Yet all too often these are insufficiently appreciated by both practitioner and patient alike.

Homoeopathy can be helpful in the prevention of epidemics. An outbreak of poliomyelitis was recently controlled by a New Zealand practitioner using *Gelsemium* with outstanding results. Other less dramatic epidemic conditions can be effectively treated or prevented using either the specific remedy or a nosode obtained from pathological material to form a no-risk vaccine. These are commonly prescribed for problems such as whooping-cough, measles, mumps, Influenza, German-measles and glandular-fever.

All the allergic problems respond well, especially asthma, eczema, urticaria and hay-fever. The latter is often best treated early in the season by specifics appropriate for the individual, before the pollen-count builds up to a level which produces severe symptoms. An autumn type of hay-fever can also occur, associated with tree moulds and for this *mixed autumn pollens* in potency may be used.

Every type of arthritis is helped by homoeopathy – osteoarthritis or rheumatism, including the degenerative conditions of aging. Common remedies prescribed include *Bryonia*, *Rhus tox*, *Medorrhinum*, *Rhododendron*, *Dulcamara*, *Apis*, *Ruta* and *Pulsatilla*. Similarly, gouty inflammations and painful conditions react positively. In some arthritic cases reported recently, where severe changes had been seen on x-ray, later films showed regeneration and new bone development in the joint area, as the remedy stimulated vitality and circulation in the region affected.

Where there is organic degeneration, especially of the liver from alcohol abuse or viral hepatitis, a return to more normal functioning can take place with *Phosphorus* in potency. This has been clearly demonstrated by improved liver-function tests when the correct specific has been used. Some continental experiments, using rats and mice, have shown that poisoned liver cells, nearly destroyed by carbon tetrachloride can clearly regenerate by being given the appropriate homoeopathic remedy. Although I do not necessarily approve of the methods and homoeopathy has been built-up over the years by clinical research on healthy human volunteers in the 'proving' experiments, nevertheless, it is of interest to see tangible proofs of the homoeopathic regenerative action.

CHAPTER ELEVEN

Preparation of the remedies

With well-tried methods, developed over many years, the homoeopathic pharmacist uses his expertise to put the basic homoeopathic substances into solution so that serial dilutions or potencies can be prepared to medicate the homoeopathic granules or tablets. The remedies are in general of plant, animal or mineral origin. Many are perfectly soluble and can be made up immediately from fresh plant tinctures with an alcohol mixture to form the mother-tincture containing pharmacologically active alkaloids. From these all other dilutions are prepared.

Some remedies are however quite insoluble in their crude form. These include minerals as phosphorous (*phosphorus*) and silica (*Silicea*) and such base metals as copper (*Cuprum*), iron (*Ferrum*), zinc (*Zincum*), lead (*Plumbum*). Hahnemann discovered an entirely new process called trituration which for the first time in medical history was able to put into solution previously insoluble sub-

115

stances. The method he used was a process of grinding-up the inert insoluble substance with sucrose and repeating the process several times until the mixture became soluble so that it became possible to create the same serial dilutions as with the soluble remedies. The use of activated salts of these substances, previously only available in their gross and less active form was in this way, finally improved upon.

In this country (U.K.), tinctures are usually diluted according to the decimal or centesimal scale, the latter being most common. Using the centesimal dilutions and the Hahnemannian method of one drop of remedy-tincture added to 99 drops of dilutant fluid, usually alcohol-based, the mixture is ready for succussing. It is vigorously shaken, traditionally about 30 times on a firm base such as a book to succuss or dynamise the substance. This forms the first centesimal potency. One drop of this in 99 drops of dilutant, again succussed, forms the second centesimal potency and so on. When the remedy has been diluted in this way six times, it becomes the sixth or 6c potency. With the decimal potencies, one drop of the remedy-tincture is diluted in 9 drops of the dilutant fluid to form the potency, again succussed at every stage. After three stages of dilution, the common potency of 3x is formed.

Standards of purity are always stringent and laid down by European pharmaceutical standards to ensure the highest degree of control and purity in the preparation of the remedies for the satisfaction of both doctor and patient. At all stages, carefully sterilised neutral glass tubes are used for the serial fluids, which are prepared by hand, up to 1000c. For the higher potencies and dilutions up to the IOM (ten thousand) and CM (one hundred thousand) a mechanical potentiser is used.

The activated tinctures are added to sucrose crystals, tablets or globules to 'hold' the remedy for use by the patient. Using a 95% water–alcohol solution for the final medication ensures that the whole of the tablets when agitated, come into contact with the chosen potency in the usual 7 gram phial prepared by the pharmacist.

It is important to realise that the remedy lies predominantly on the surface or outside of the pill or tablet used. For this reason they should not be handled when taken and one only shaken into their container lid and crushed or swallowed on the tongue. In particular no remedy should be handled for another person when prescibed. They should always be taken well away from food, tea or coffee and stored in a clean glass jar, preferably a new one, not near any perfumed items as soaps, perfumes, herbs or spices. The container should not have been used previously for other medicines – either allopathic or homoeopathic, as there is a risk of neutralising or contaminating the remedies and making them ineffective.

There is another method of preparing the potencies which finds favour on the continent although less so here in the U.K. This is also an early method which does not use serial tubes but relies upon a single container where the 99 to one ratio is strictly kept to, but where one drop is considered to adhere to the inside of the container after succussing. In this Korsakov method, the dilutant fiuid

117

is thrown out of the same jar each time after succussion and a further 99 drops added each time to complete the serial ratios. The same bottle is used for each potency until the required one is achieved.

Note that all the 'finished' remedies look, taste, and smell alike and cannot be differentiated by cyrstallography or chromatography methods at this stage in our knowledge. Research is continuing to differentiate the potencies by electronic spectrum methods.

In the U.K. many practitioners follow the guide-lines laid down by the great American homoeopath Kent who recommended taking only the single remedy at a time and continuing with that remedy for as long as it is benefiting the patient and there is a healing response and improvement. He recommended a change of remedy only when improvement stopped or there was no reaction of a dynamic kind to the potency given or simply when nothing happened. When symptoms abate and are completely cleared, then the remedy should be omitted completely and the patient take nothing at all, letting the body's natural defences and vitality 'take the wheel'.

CHAPTER TWELVE

Making a start

The first step always seems the longest and most difficult and so it may appear in homoeopathy too – but the method is not complicated, and the principles once grasped are simple and logical. To familiarise yourself with the method nevertheless takes a period of time, to gain confidence in the new approach and the remedies. To obtain this experience it is advisable to begin with the following four simplest remedies from the twenty listed and recommended in chapter twenty. Begin with remedies in the 6th centesimal or 6c potency and start as outlined below. Always buy your remedies from an established and preferably recommended pharmacy, but in all cases get to know your pharmacist. The source of your remedies must be of the highest quality at all times.

Arnica is the most commonly prescribed remedy of all, probably the most useful and basic for the beginner. Use it in any situation of painful bruising and swelling after trauma – for example from a fall or tumble, a heavy knock or any similar cause. It is invaluable for psychological hurts and shocks as well as the physical ones. Sometimes there is the quite spontaneous development of 'bruised', left-sided pain in a rib or costal muscle, occurring after strain in that region – from carrying the unaccustomed weight of a heavy suitcase or for some reason as changing from an electric typewriter to a manual one. What is important in the choice of *Arnica* as the indicated remedy is the quality of the bruised and swollen feeling in the area affected. Muscular strain responds well, as after lifting a heavy weight and being suddenly caught off-balance. The unaccustomed use of a ladder – in late summer for fruit-picking, when winter-pruning, or decorating the home can also cause pain and a bruised aching situation – just the type of pain for *Arnica* which gives rapid relief. Any situation that puts strain on unusual areas of tendon and muscle leading to pain or an actual bruise developing is when the remedy is most valuable. For a very painful condition it may be given hourly but with the majority of conditions, three times a day is adequate.

Aconitum is the greatest remedy for fear reactions of any kind especially acute ones. It is valuable for sudden chill from exposure to an East wind or from cold and draughts. Neuralgic pains often occur as a result of such exposures, and provided they are caught within the first 48 hours by the remedy, such painful conditions are quickly resolved. There may be an acute headache, or a sore throat from a cold with pains in the scalp, neck and facial area. *Aconitum* is of help for reactions of acute shock, especially those of fear, fright or panic – the person caught psychologically off-balance and unprepared at the time, leading to agitation and restlessness. In these conditions of either physical or psychological exposure, then *Aconitum* is invaluable. Always use the remedy as early as possible, especially during the first 48 hours after exposure – whatever its cause – you will find that given the correct indications, *Aconitum* gives quick and almost immediate results.

Calendula is unique in stimulating healthy healing and the formation of granulation tissue to protect and cover a wound or cut. A severe wound needs suturing. One acutely infected, or where there is foreign matter within the lesion requires treatment in the nearest casualty department. But *Calendula* can still be safely given in the 6th potency internally and also applied locally as a tincture when generally cleaning the area. Use it for all cuts, abrasions and wounds. Its power to stimulate healing is often astonishing.

The marigold plant in tincture has remarkable healing properties when used internally, or applied locally. It is of particular value for open cuts, wounds and scratches, lesions of any kind where there is pain, discharge and soreness. It stimulates the formation of granulation and scar tissue and has healing properties where there has been a superficial burn or scald. It is also useful for the treatment of dry eczemas and erysipelas.

Calendula can be safety given internally, in the 6th or 30c potencies, to stimulate healing and to minimise the spread of infection. It should be routine treatment for all small cuts, abrasions and wounds in the home at every age and whenever there is a need for first aid.

Rhus Tox is indicated for conditions of muscular or tendon strain where there is a spasmodic aching or painful conditions such as lumbago, from exposure to cold and damp, or sudden strain from cold air on an area of 'pulled' muscle; especially where sweating has made the area vulnerable to cooling and chill. Sprains, strain, any form of muscular swelling with tenderness, – frequently from trauma indicates *Rhus tox*. It often follows *Arnica* and is also useful for itchy, red, eczematous conditions with a limited local or small areas of eruption. In all cases when the remedy is indicated the condition is usually better for warmth, often local heat and generally made worse by cold air and damp. Movement rather than immobility gives relief and comfort so that the patient tends to move a lot or to fidget, wanting to be up and about, rather than resting in bed or sitting in a chair. This motion gives relief from tension and any spasm present.

Nux vomica is basic to every home first-aid kit and should be studied early because of its wide value. Like *Calendula* it can be used for every age group of the family. Its key notes are pain, spasm and irritability, whether these occur either physically or psychologically. Nausea is usually associated and *Nux vom* can be used when there is a combination of sickness and irritability of emotional origin or for nausea, spasm and an irritable stomach following dietary indiscretion. It is useful for pain and cramps in any part of the body – a tension headache, acute lumbago, menstrual pain or period colic. Any irritable condition may be helped by *Nux vomica* – from the irritability of a small child who is teething where *Chamomilla* has not been totally curative – to the tension of the anxious, tired executive, worried about promotion or redundancy. In a similar way, the irritability of a tired mum, not getting enough help and support with the housework and young children is also often helped by *Nux vomica* or *Sepia*.

Start to think homoeopathically in your overall general approach to a problem, one which you intend to treat yourself. Don't just think of treating a 'cold' or 'headache', but rather think of the person and overall type of problem and complaint rather than quickly giving a name to it. This 'naming' is more of a barrier to homoeopathy than an aid. Jot down the symptoms – the things complained of by the individual. Try to see clearly the type of head-cold for example which is distressing. If there are three children in the family, all down with a cold, almost certainly each one will have a slightly different and varying symptom-pattern. Note how the cold came on and anything that caused or aggravated it. Also note anything that is especially desired or disliked – a craving for hot drinks (*Arsenicum*) or ice-cold ones (*Phosphorus*). Some patients have an intense, almost obsessional dislike of the least draught or cool air because it aggravates their condition, yet others crave fresh air and want all the doors and windows

123

open (*Pulsatilla*).

Note too the colour, pattern and characteristics of any discharge occurring. A nasal discharge may be continuous, thin and watery (*Allium cepa*) or it may be yellow, greenish, thick and full of mucus (*Kali bich*). Some excretions are excoriating, burning to neighbouring tissues causing pain and discomfort. With others the discharge is more dry and stringy (*Hydrastis*). In general note the factors which make the condition worse and the time of day when symptoms are most severe as well as eased – for example in the morning, or better at the end of the day.

All of this gives an overall viewpoint and helps ensure that the correct remedy is chosen for the particular individual's needs at the time. The more accurate the prescription, the more efficient the remedy. An approximate, close-fitting remedy may give a degree of symptom relief but is unlikely to affect a cure. Some relief may occur, but the results are often disappointing to both patient and prescriber – in many cases blaming the method rather than inaccurate prescribing. In general – approximately is not good enough for homoeopathy and a lasting cure. So make sure of this overall way of looking and thinking, then you can be sure of far better results on each occasion. Try to make this broader looking, thinking and approach to homoeopathic prescribing a discipline so that you can gradually learn with experience more and more of the responses to the remedies, their characteristics, and build on this experience. Especially gain skill by practise initially, using the twenty basic remedies so that your results and ability-to-prescribe is assured with increasing certainty and confidence.

When learning to familiarise yourself with the common remedies always be aware of laterality – or the side of the body affected. Note whether a tonsillar infection is predominantly left or right-sided, or a lumbago, painful knee, or gouty condition and note too if the condition commenced on one side and then later moved over to involve the other half of the body. The laterality of major remedies must be known, those which are primarily right-sided as where the action is mainly on the left part of the body.

Right-sided remedies include: *Lycopodium, Bryonia, Belladonna, Nux vom.*

Left-sided remedies include: *Lachesis, Kali carb, Graphites, Sepia, Sulphur.*

The key psychological aspects of the basic remedies must also be clearly known as this is indispensable to good and accurate prescribing. The major 'mentals' include:

The irritability of *Nux vom*
The fear of *Aconitum*
The indifference of *Sepia*
The pride of *Platina*
The jealousy of *Lachesis*
The resentment of *Staphisagria*
The passivity and tearfulness of *Pulsatilla*

Try to get quite clear the distinguishing mobility

factors of each major remedy you are using and working are on, such as:

The restless and agitation of *Rhus tox*, *Arsenicum*, *Zincum met*.

The immobility of *Bryonia*.

The other factors to be quite clear about and which may 'make' or clinch the diagnosis are

Thirst – absent in *Pulsatilla*, *Apis*

Thirst – frequent in *Calcarea* and *Phosphorus* (for ice-cold drinks).

Note whether the patient is sweating or not and if the perspiration is offensive.

Absence of sweating – *Lycopodium*.

Profuse sweating – *Calcarea* (particularly of the forehead), *Thuja* (generalised, sweetish and strong), *Mercurius* (offensive), *Ipecacuanha* (associated with nausea and excessive salivation), *Silicea* (on covered areas).

The general metabolism and heat output of both patient and remedy should be known in order to make an accurate choice of prescription.

For example *Belladonna*, *Sulphur* – both burning hot.

Arsenicum, *Silicea* and *Calcarea* always very cold and chilly, craving heat.

Pulsatilla is chilly and cold but intolerant of the least warmth.

CHAPTER THIRTEEN

Homoeopathy and the home

Don't be tempted to regard homoeopathy as a panacea, nor become a martyr to it, using it as an act of faith, religion or as an outlet for spiritual needs. When homoeopathy becomes an article of faith rather than a scientific instrument it is in danger of becoming an obsession which can only undermine its value. It is important to keep a balance in all things and no one should go 'overboard' over homoeopathy. It should be used in a non-emotional way as a non-mystical medical treatment. For others, homoeopathy only has priority of treatment when the conventional approaches have failed – from lack of knowledge of its therapeutic power.

A holistic approach is implicit to homoeopathy which does not deny or exclude either the scientific or the new, provided that they are necessary, indicated and do not constitute a risk for the patient, or a purely experimental approach. Where the dangers, risks and side-effects of a dubious treat-

127

ment outweigh the gains for the patient, then homoeopathy gives a safer, better response for the person in his totality.

Homoeopathy has never been a second-class citizen in the treatment stakes and many families have used homoeopathy effectively for varied conditions over several generations. It is a well-tried first-line treatment approach. Some only use homoeopathy however when conventional treatments are unsatisfactory after frequent trials. In many ways this is a wrong use of homoeopathy because such methods have too often depleted and jaded the patient beyond all limits, quite separately from any diminishing effects from their illness. Under such conditions, homoeopathy is slower to act because of a depleted sluggish vitality from drug side-effects, which may take weeks or months to recover from or to remove from the system.

Because of its overall effectiveness, in so many areas, there is no reason why homoeopathy should not be used as the front-line approach to illness. The method can be curative at all ages, naturally depending upon the type of constitution and condition treated, its severity and duration. In the child, the remedies can be used preventatively for all the major childhood conditions where there is a special risk as with severe outbreaks of measles, whooping-cough, chicken pox and mumps – using the nosode or homoeopathic vaccine-equivalent without the increasingly recognized risks of conventional vaccination.

It is helpful with young babies for teething problems or where there is wind or digestive discomfort. In the nursing mother many of the common feeding problems which occur – such as soreness of breast or nipple can be quickly dealt with and eased. Childhood complaints of eczema and asthma, the common infective illnesses, a sore throat, hay-fever, allergic rhinitis with a continual blocked nose or ear problem not responding to ever-changing antibiotic after antibiotic, can be treated by homoeopathy.

Chronic conditions of both child and adolescent like acne, rheumatoid arthritis or tonsillitis, are also within the curative range of the well-chosen remedy. The common adult problems of peptic ulcer, hiatus hernia, blood-pressure, angina of effort usually respond well and long periods of pain and discomfort relieved. Menstrual problems with hot flushes, drenching sweats, period pains and premenstrual tension are daily treated by homoeopathy with good results.

The elderly have their own areas of particular problem which respond, given good-will and patience. The commonest difficulties are the arthritic ones, seen at all ages and in all degrees. Prostatic problems, or those of bladder weakness and prolapse are also common. All these problems can show a positive noticeable response to homoepathic treatment and quite frequently improvement occurs without a long pause or delay.

When there is an overwhelming problem of meningitis, pneumonia, influenza of the elderly, appendicitis, collapse, stroke, any form of severe haemorrhage or severe infection where antibiotics are valuable and well and truly indicated, then homoeopathy should only be used to support the patient until the doctor comes or until he is moved

129

to hospital. Both *Arnica* and the Bach rescue remedy drops are invaluable. Such methods effectively help to relieve shock and moreover act as a valuable often essential supportive therapy to conventional treatments and surgery when required.

Stress illness of the adult or child in any form responds well and quickly to the potencies when carefully chosen and treated early. Homoeopathy can give a rapid resolution to many acute problems and a quick return to a more relaxed and balanced self. If the problem is an overwhelming one or due to severe shock, then more time for healing must obviously be expected and allowed for in every case.

I have already mentioned the nosodes in the prevention of childhood illness but they also have a role where an adult is especially vulnerable or at risk. I am thinking particularly of such exposures as an adult male in contact with the child with mumps, where the adult has no natural immunity from a previous childhood infection. Orchitis and possible sterility is a real risk and the specific nosode gives welcome protection. Similarly the early pregnant mother must be protected from all contacts and risks of infection with rubella or German measles – indeed any viral illness – during the early weeks of pregnancy. The rubella nosode is useful prophylactically where a suspected contact may have unwittingly occurred or only discovered in retrospect. In an elderly person too who is convalescent and especially vulnerable, where influenza is a possibility, or there is a history of earlier chronic bronchitis or emphysema, then the influenza nosode may be given to protect and

130

lessen the impact of any infection that does occur. In this way the risks of complications occurring in an already vulnerable and weakened constitution are reduced.

Chronic problems, especially the psychological ones respond well to homoeopathy but it is also of value in certain more physical and mechanical conditions if surgery is either undesirable or impossible or where it has failed for a variety of reasons. In such cases – for example of hiatus hernia, prolapse, rupture (hernia), these may respond well in terms of symptom-relief even where the mechanical problem is not markedly changed. I have frequently had good results with uterine prolapse of the elderly where over a period of months the prolapse has no longer 'come down' as before homoeopathic treatment.

In all cases, should a prolapse or hernia become twisted upon itself, strangulated or irreducible, so that the blood supply is cut-off, then surgery is immediately indicated whatever the state of general health.

Homoeopathy should never be used as an alternative to surgery in cases of appendicitis or where it is suspected and a surgical opinion must always be sought at any age. In general the best treatment of all disease and illness is prevention and early diagnosis. Especially where there is a problem of severe organic disease or cancer, the most modern proved techniques may be combined with traditional homoeopathic ones – as a secondary back-up or when conventional treatment has failed or is no longer indicated. At such times homoeopathy can be used as the total approach in a variety of

131

potencies as best fits the symptoms and the patterns of organic dysfunction caused by the disease.

Homoeopathy, as with any form of treatment, however advantageous, has both its advantages and its limitations. There are periods when homoeopathy must be used in the background. However enthusiastic you may be, don't prescribe homoeopathy for a problem that requires surgery or a traditional approach. When in doubt ask your doctor, get a consultation and proper professional advice.

Homoeopathy implies a totality of overall approach and viewpoint which should not be dogmatic or rigid. Your flexibility of mind is most important. There is no need to try and create magic with homoeopathy – the method just does not need it and this is not how it is meant to be used. There are specific indications for homoeopathy and when these are not present then another method should be used or considered. In the final diagnosis it is always the patient who matters most of all and not the principles or method of cure however much you are in favour of them. A particular approach – even a homoeopathic one must be right for the individual patient – if not it will fail as it is no longer holistic.

CHAPTER FOURTEEN

First Aid

Cuts and wounds

Clean the area very carefully with *Calendula* lotion, removing foreign material of any kind which is present. All bleeding must be stopped by local pressure in the area using clean gauze or cotton wool. If a tourniquet is used, it must be released frequently. When the wound is severe give *Arnica 6* for shock hourly or the Bach rescue remedy, 5 drops to be repeated hourly until shock (collapse) is no longer present. Keep the patient warm and covered whenever the patient is in shock and give warm drinks. *Calendula* should be applied both locally to the wound area and given internally in the 6th potency hourly for the first few hours and then three times daily. Honey is often a useful local dressing to apply as an alternative to calendula and the dressing need not be removed for several days before being replaced by a similar one. *Hypericum* is indicated in the 6th potency whenever there is damage to nerve tissue with bruising or shooting nerve pains going up the limbs from the hand or foot. When the wound involves tendons, *Ruta* or *Bellis perennis* should be used as soon as the initial shock period has passed. If the area involved is muscle, give *Rhus tox* 6 and when the main area affected is bone or periosteum – the fine tissue sheath covering the bones – give *Symphytum* 6 three times daily.

Foreign bodies

Essentially these are irritants to local tissue and must always be removed to avoid a severe infective reaction. They may occur in any of the orifices of the body including the eyes and must be removed gently with care to avoid damage to the delicate tissues in the area. A protective inflammatory reaction usually occurs almost immediately. Having removed the object from the nostril, ear, eye, or on occasions genital area, apply *Calendula* locally if there are any signs of an inflammatory-reaction, and give either *Calendula 6* internally three times daily for three days or use *Arnica* if there is evidence of marked swelling or bruising in the area.

Black Eye

Due to a blow or injury. Initial treatment should be *Arnica 30* for shock repeated hourly until there is an improvement. When there has been an acute or severe fear reaction give *Aconitum 6* three times daily for three days. *Ledum* (Marsh tea) is an excellent remedy when the areas are red rather than black, the patient chilly and cold, often in a

134

cold sweat. They may be improved by a local cold compress to the area affected. *Hamamelis 6* is of value when the haemorrhagic area is darker and blacker than with the *Ledum* type of eye. Use *Ruta* (Rue) in the 6th potency when there is much pain in the area from bruising of bone causing discomfort. If the eyeball itself is affected and painful use *Symphytum 6* three times daily and if it persists a specialist unit should be consulted to exclude any damage to the eye which may require surgical or other specialised treatment.

Falls and sprains

The major immediate remedy should be *Arnica 6* for swelling and bruising to tissues in the area. *Hypericum* is useful for pain of bruised and stretched delicate nervous tissue which is often associated, or when there are shooting pains. In general a firm supportive bandage is recommended, often a cold application to the part to reduce swelling. *Ruta* is indicated for tendon and bone pain or tenderness. Use *Rhus tox* when there is residual muscular stiffness, better for heat. If there is severe pain in the area, aggravated by the least movement, *Bryonia* is indicated. *Belladonna* is only useful when the area is red and congested, sensitive to the least movement or jarring sensation. *Bellis perennis* is a fine remedy where there is swelling and pain from sprain, worsened and aggravated by damp or cold with marked weakness and exhaustion and a need to lie down. Recurrent sprains, especially of the ankles might indicate *Calcarea* if there is a chilly disposition and weakness with obesity. For a tendency to accident-proneness generally, with sprain part of an overall self-destructive pattern, consider *Kali carb* as the remedy of choice.

Puncture wounds from bites and stings

As always in homoeopathy, the remedy depends upon the symptom-picture. When there has been a simple puncture-wound which is clean and uncomplicated, as from a cat-bite or other small animal, then the best remedy is *Ledum 6* three times daily. When there is pain and swelling use *Calendula* locally or *Hypericum* when the pain is severe and shooting in character. For a bee sting use *Apis 6* and for a painful wasp sting – either *Arnica* or *Rhus tox* – the latter when there is considerable redness and irritation. If the area affected is very swollen and irritating with blister formation after a bite – as occurs with an allergic reaction, use *Urtica 6* hourly if severe, or three times daily if less so. Should the reaction to a bite or sting be very severe, with redness and inflammation spreading up the arm or leg, use *Belladonna* 6. When the area is dark red, swollen and painful, with a blue discolouration, and intolerance of pressure or covering to the area, give *Lachesis* 6 hourly until there is relief. After a snake bite, try to remove the venom by sucking the area and spitting out afterwards. The patient should be removed to hospital at the earliest opportunity. Give *Arnica* 6 or 30c for shock. When the patient is ice-cold and collapsing give *Carbo veg.* instead of *Arnica* to revive.

Nose Bleeding (epistaxis)

These are common in many children and occur quite spontaneously or are associated with agitation and restlessness. In the adult it may be a sign of raised blood-pressure when recurrent and it is generally a good indication to have a complete physical check-up. Use simple local pressure or packing of the nostril to control the bleeding. *Hamamelis* (Witch hazel) is the most useful remedy for recurrent conditions in the child. When the cause is from a fall or tumble use *Arnica* 6 hourly until there is relief. If the cause is more emotional, give *Ignatia* where associated with tears or loss in any form. Use *Natrum mur* for a more generalised emotional disturbance. When associated with fainting and heat give *Pulsatilla 6*.

Bruises

Bruises are usually the result of a simple traumatic happening with localised blueness and swelling. In general *Arnica* covers the majority of cases and there is rapid relief. If not, consider *Bellis perennis* (the common daisy) for cases associated with pain, swelling and feeling exhausted. In some instances the bruising is quite spontaneous and independent of any injury. For such cases consider *Phosphorus* and if recurrent, a check-up and blood profile is recommended to clarify the causes of any bleeding-tendency into the skin or nearby tissues.

Hiccough

The common condition of recurrent brief spasmodic contractions of the diaphragm, usually digestive in origin. Most cases respond well and quickly to *Nux vom* 6 given every ten minutes until there is relief. When associated with an emotional upset *Natrum mur.* is preferable in the 30th potency and repeated after half an hour if there is no relief. *Arsenicum* can be used when there is a sudden chill and shivering. Use *Pulsatilla* where the condition is linked to a child or adult getting over-heated and exhausted, often after tears.

Other remedies which need to be considered include *Ginseng* – where the hiccough is associated with low back pain or sciatica; *Ratanhia* – for violent hiccough with strong rectal discomfort – as if containing broken glass; *Sulph. ac* – when there is considerable associated weakness, perspiration and trembling.

Fainting

This is another common 'household emergency', and it can be often quite worrying to onlookers when a faint is severe. The commonest cause is a hot and airless situation when *Pulsatilla* usually gives a quick response. The best general remedy to use is the Bach rescue drops as an immediate emergency measure, 5 drops on the tongue. When due to weakness and exhaustion use *China* 6. If caused by emotion at the sight of blood give *Nux. vomica*. Where the patient is cold, marble-white, chilly and covered with sweat give *Carbo veg* or

138

Veratrum alb. Fainting from fear needs *Aconitum* to correct it. When associated with prolonged standing and immobility give *Alumina 30*.

Diarrhoea

This is a frequent problem for both adult and child. It is most dangerous in the young baby because of the risks of dehydration. In this age group treatment is best given by a physician. There are many possible remedies available and they need to be carefully differentiated by the overall condition as well as the characteristics of the stool. A watery unformed stool may require *Sulphur*, *Podophyllum*, *Nux vom* or *Mercurius*. Where the stool is more varied, *Pulsatilla* may be needed. If blood is present *Phosphorus* or *Hamamelis* may be required and a green stool is often an indication for *Chamomilla*. A pale watery stool suggests *Calcarea* a more yellow stool *Chelidonium*. In all these diarrhoeal problems the general state gives the clue to the appropriate remedy when prescribing. Any suggestion of dehydration, shock or collapse may require immediate hospitalisation.

Vomiting

One of the most common household emergencies. Try to ascertain the cause whatever the age of the person and be especially careful in an adult or child where the problem is repetitive or relatively 'out of keeping' with the person. For the vomiting of pregnancy consider *Kreosotum*, *Tabacum* or *Nux vom*. Important general remedies for vomiting

139

include *Aconitum*, *Lobelia*, *Nux vom*, *Arsenicum*, *Antimonium tart*. Try and get a clear picture of the pattern of vomiting, any aggravating factors and its overall taste, colour and frequency. Note also the key times and relate these to the remedy. For example, early morning suggests *Hepar sulph*; mid-morning sickness – *Psorinum*; Noon vomiting – *Mag. carb*.; afternoon problems – *Sulphur*; evening sickness – *Carbo Veg*; late night-time vomiting includes remedies as *Calcarea* or *Ferrum met*.

Toothache

The most valuable general remedies are *Coffea*, *Chamomilla*, *Staphisagria*, *China*, *Belladonna*, *Hepar sulph*. All of these should be known and differentiated. It is not the purpose of this present volume to deal with the remedies in detail, but each one has its appropriate site of pain, type and time of aggravation which is important for accurate prescribing. Also of value are *Plantago* – where there is salivation and the teeth feel 'too long', pain worse for the least pressure or touch; *Magnesia carb* – toothache of a tearing kind especially useful during pregnancy – the breath has a sour odour.

Indigestion and flatulence

Major general remedies include *Argentum nit*, *Lycopodium*, *Nux vom*, and these should be familiar to the prescriber. Indigestion on waking may indicate *Sulphur* or *Lachesis*. Morning problems often respond well to *Baptisia* whilst afternoon dyspepsia with flatulence, about 4.00 p.m.

responds best to *Lycopodium*. Late evening indigestion often indicates *Pulsatilla* when the general features fit the remedy. Where symptoms occur in the early hours, about 3 to 5.00 a.m. then the remedy is more likely to be *Kali carb*. For general flatulence and discomfort, *Cargo veg*. is highly dependable. In all cases, a careful overall look at the person must be made, especially for 'first time' indigestion or any change of eating-patterns in the adult. Also any loss of appetite or weight-loss, inexplicable general malaise, with odd or bizarre symptoms is an indication for a full professional check-up. When symptoms persist, fail to respond, or get worse with homoeopathy, this is also an indication for a full physical examination, especially when a seemingly well-prescribed and well-indicated remedy has been given. If the response to prescribing is at all poor or disappointing, there may be an underlying organic lesion, which makes a homoeopathic response impossible or short-lasting. All of these features indicate a medical check-up. An alternative to this professional examination is a check-up at one of the diagnostic centres which several of the private insurance companies make generally available, the results sent to the patient's general practitioner. In this way a stress problem or one of simple dysfunction and a temporary matter, can be differentiated from any more serious underlying organic disease which may require a different or additional treatment to the homoeopathic one.

Temperature

In all cases where there is a raised temperature above the normal of 98.4 F or 37 C, the cause should be ascertained. Usually the reason is an infection somewhere or other – perhaps of the ear, sinuses, throat, teeth or due to a common cold. But there are exceptions and a stress illness can equally produce a temperature. Remedies include *Hepar sulph*, *Belladonna*, *Pyrogen*, *Mercurius*, *Aconitum*, *Phytolacca*. The site of infection, side of throat or ear infected is relevant to the remedy chosen. Also the degree of sweating, restlessness, pain and psychological attitudes are important in choosing the right remedy. When well-chosen, the results are often dramatic. In most cases, the patient is best kept in bed, and given fluids only until the temperature subsides. When a raised temperature heralds one of the more general childhood infective illnesses, then the specific nosode of that disease may be required as well as one of the above. The child may also have to be kept isolated from others for a time during the acute infective period.

Hang-over

Strictly speaking a 'hair of the dog' is homoeopathic and perhaps the reason for its popularity with many alcoholics on waking and before they can begin their day. In general however it is not recommended because it simply reinforces the habit and a remedy that provokes *similar*, but not exactly identical symptoms is preferable. *Avena sat.* (oats) is highly recommended by many, but I prefer either *Nux vom* or *Sulphur* for such morn-

142

ing symptoms combined with a high natural vitamin dietary regime. Vitamin *B* in potency gives improved results and supports homoeopathic treatment.

Headache

Where the pain is over the forehead, of a dull heavy nature, then *Bryonia* or *Belladonna* is useful. Pain at the back of the head in the occipital region responds to *Nux vom* or *Carbo veg* and especially *Silicea* where it has moved backwards from the forehead region and settled in the occiput.

Pain in the temples is often helped by *Natrum mur*. If the headache increases in severity or the back of the neck is stiff and there is high fever, the diagnosis of meningitis must be excluded by a doctor as soon as possible and hospitalisation arranged if at all likely. A small haemorrhage or leakage from a cerebral aneurysm can also cause similar symptoms with irritability, particularly in young adults. Where symptoms fail to respond or are getting worse, then get a medical opinion as soon as possible. In this latter case a lumbar puncture may be essential to reduce intracranial pressure and to relieve headache. Most cases however are of the simple migraine kind and there is a good response to the homoeopathic prescription calming agitation and giving relief of pain. Only when there is no response should a family be on their guard and think of alternative diagnosis where the correct approach may not be homoeopathy but hospitalisation with conventional investigation and treatments.

143

Colic

The type of pain, time of day or night and area affected are all relevant to finding the right remedy. For colic pain which bends the patient double, consider *Mag. phos*, *Colocynth*, *Belladonna*, *Pulsatilla*, *Graphites*, or *Chamomilla*. All of these have their distinct diagnostic features, laterality and distinguishing hallmarks which help decide the best remedy. Where colic is associated with flatulence then consider either *Nux vom* – especially where irritability is marked, or *Carbo veg*.

Sea-sickness

The best remedies are often *Tabacum*, *Cocculus*, *Kali carb*, or *Petroleum*. Each must be differentiated according to the particular symptoms, degree of problem and the amount of sweating, collapse, mucus production and vertigo present.

Petroleum is a most valuable remedy, when there is marked salivation, vertigo on rising from the prone position, and sour eructations with vomiting and marked hunger; *Cocculus* – is also helpful for faintness and vomiting, but in contrast to the *Petroleum* remedy, there is loss of interest in food and abdominal pain – the abdomen has a 'hollow' feeling. *Pulsatilla* – is indicated for acute conditions with a bitter taste, flatulence, intolerance of heat and the absence of thirst. *Natrum mur* has weakness and exhaustion as one of its key notes with sweating, heartburn, stomach pains, tearfulness, thirst, anxiety and restlessness. *Nux vomica* is for a combination of gastric spasm, irritability,

144

flatulence and hypersensitivity to noise and bright lights or the least pressure on the stomach.

Acute throat conditions

One of the most common household first-aid emergencies, especially among school children, when every few weeks a vulnerable child can miss school because of the recurrent illness with high temperature and sore throat. The lymph nodes are often tender and swollen with loss of appetite and energy. Repeated antibiotics, seem to be of no real assistance and only undermine further the child's natural immune resistance. Many parents turn in desperation to homoeopathy after yet another antibiotic has done nothing for the child. The homoeopathic response is often encouraging and major remedies include *Belladonna*, *Phytolacca*, *Causticum*, *Sulphur*, *Hepar sulph*, *Nitric acid* and *Mercurius*. Where the problem is definitely worse on one side, consider *Lachesis* for left-sided tonsillar infections when raw and tender and *Lycopodium* for a right-sided problem. For suppuration or definite pus formation give either *Silicea* or *Mercurius* – especially for abscess formation (quinsy) in the tonsillar area. If the condition worsens, and there is the least indication of difficult or obstructed breathing, call an ambulance and send the child to hospital immediately.

Acute ear problems

Belladonna is often the best remedy, or *Pulsatilla* for a less severe and less 'hot' type of problem with

145

more variable and changeable characteristics. *Chamomilla* is indicated for very severe pain, but both *Phosphorus* and *Hepar sulph* are also useful. Make sure that there is not a foreign body in the ear causing blockage and infection. If in doubt, or it cannot be easily removed, call for expert professional help. In general right-sided acute ear problems respond well to *Belladonna* or *Fluoric acid* and left-sided infections more to *Aconitum*, *Graphites* or *Dulcamara*.

Sleeplessness

When there is inability to get off to sleep from an over-active mind then *Lycopodium* is helpful. But where insomnia occurs in the early morning hours, waking about 5.00 a.m. with restless vague anxiety, often *Kali carb*. is more indicated. Sudden waking with fear and agitation at about midnight or just after, especially with a feeling of chill, indicates *Arsenicum*. Where wakefulness occurs a little later, about 2–3.00 a.m., this time with a sense of heat, the need to pass water, to throw off the covers, or push the feet out, but no sooner out then freezing cold, the remedy is *Pulsatilla*. Another useful general remedy, for tension, agitation and restlessness is *Coffea*. More general wakefulness from anxiety and vague apprehension may need *Natrum mur*. If the underlying problem is one of fear and grave insecurity then consider *Aconitum* as the remedy of choice. *Ignatia* is indicated for insomnia of the recently widowed and where grief and mourning are major factors.

Lack of natural sleep often results from abuse of

sedative drugs over a long period which have eroded sleep patterns. Everyone needs sleep for essential rest and when it is undermined the underlying causes must be clearly ascertained and corrected. The use and dependency upon artificial sedatives is best removed slowly so that sleep can again take on more natural patterns as the homoeopathic remedy restores rest and relaxation.

Remedies to consider include *Lycopodium* – where there is difficulty in going to sleep because of an over-active mind or fears about the future. *Arsenicum* – when the person wakes just after midnight, about 1.00 a.m, especially associated with chill and poor circulation. *Kali carb* – for early waking between 3.00 and 5.00 a.m., falling asleep exhausted, just before the alarm rings with vague restless anxiety. *Nux vomica* – after a dietary indiscretion or from an excessive ill-balanced meal. *Coffea* – where there has been abuse of tea or coffee over a prolonged period with build-up of tension, agitation and restlessness.

Lumbago

Remedies include *Rhus tox*, *Bryonia*, *Rhododendron*, *Nux vom*, *Dulcamara*. Each has its specific and distinctive type of symptomatology which should be known. The cause is also important – either from strain (*Rhus tox*); exposure to damp (*Pulsatilla*); due to a change of weather (*Dulcamara*); exposure to a cold dry wind (*Bryonia*); associated with period and uterine problems, the pains felt in the low back region (*Sepia*). Some forms of lumbago are markedly relieved by heat

147

and rubbing (*Rhus tox*) yet others are not helped at all or even worsened (*Bryonia*). Where the discomfort need firm local support and pressure to obtain relief from pain, *Natrum mur.* should be considered.

The Common Cold

The best remedy at an early stage is often *Aconitum*, if the condition can be caught within the first 48 hours. Following this I recommend either *Nux vomica*, *Arsenicum* or *Gelsemium*, depending upon the symptom-pattern of the individual, the degree of chilliness or weakness. Where there is a 'flu' epidemic in the area, consider the specific nosode *Influenzinum*. For severe blocked nasal congestion give *Kali bich.* or *Kali carb.* and where the discharge is green, yellow or variable, use *Pulsatilla*. A continuous watery, drip-discharge may need *Allium cepa* for relief. If the temperature is raised consider *Hepar sulph*. In general keep the patient on fluids until the fever subsides.

Boils

Boils are the common localised infection of the skin with pus formation, redness and severe lancing pain. *Belladonna* is best for the acute stage and followed by *Sulphur* if the condition persists. Where there is an associated toxic condition or raised temperature, think of *Mercurius* or possibly *Hepar sulph*. Should the condition worsen, enlarge and discharge frank pus or form a deep crater, becoming a carbuncle, then *Anthracinum* is more

148

the remedy of choice, followed by *Silicea* or *Arsenicum*.

Breathlessness

This is an important condition and it is necessary to get the diagnosis right. If in doubt do not hesitate to get medical advice. Where recurrent asthma is the reason, major remedies include *Medorrhinium*, *Phosphorus*, *Natrum mur*, *Arsenicum* or *Ipecacuanha*. Chronic bronchitis may require *Sulphur* or *Kali carb*. The time of onset of the attack is important. For morning breathlessness – *Sulphur* or *Sepia*; for onset in the early afternoon – *China.*; for evening breathing difficulties – consider *Pulsatilla* or *Lycopodium*. After midnight *Arsenicum* may be required. In the early morning hours think of *Ammonium mur* or *Kali carb*. Where due to anger remember *Nux vom*; damp – *Dulcamara*; from an emotional outburst – *Natrum mur*; exposure to chill – *Apis*; from a heat reaction – *Pulsatilla*.

CHAPTER FIFTEEN

The twenty basic remedies and their usage

The recommended basic remedies for the family homoeopathic chest are – *Aconitum, Arnica, Arsenicum alb., Belladonna, Bryonia, Carbo veg, Chamomilla, Gelsemium, Heparsulph, Hypericum, Kali bic, Ledum, Lycopodium, Mag phos., Natrum mur, Nux vom, Sepia, Sulphur, Thuja.*

Aconitum (Monkshood)

This is the most acute of all remedies and most efficient when given within the first 48 hours of onset of symptoms. There is a mixture of fear, anxiety, uncertainty and agitation, often with pain, diarrhoea or headache. The commonest causative factors for the typically painful and inflammatory condition are chill from cold or damp air. Often a seemingly strong, healthy-looking person, well-built and active is struck-down by acute bronchitis, or an alimentary infection. They are convinced that death is imminent. All symptoms are aggravated by heat, the bed coverings and at midnight. Where an illness is clearly the result of fear give *Aconitum* in the 30th potency even if many years have elapsed since the original fright. The remedy is particularly useful in acute chest conditions especially when associated with pleurisy and severe pain in the side on coughing or the least sudden movement (*Bryonia*).

Arnica (Leopards Bane)

Arnica is a remedy for soft-tissue injury with haemorrhage into the tissues and swelling from haematoma or the accumulation of blood under the skin. The area is black and blue with general weakness and a sore bruised feeling. The psychological disposition is vulnerability and the person feels hurt, fearful and anxious wanting to be left as quiet as possible. It is the greatest of all remedies and most easy to use, so that it is ideally suited for the beginner to homoeopathy. Pain and swelling with bruising is the key to *Arnica* and shock of either an emotional or traumatic cause, with damage to tissues. It is indicated both pre- and post-operatively or during the convalescent period. Also for dental interventions and after loss of blood with shock and weakness. The *Arnica* personality is typically sensitive, but also physically too so that they are intolerant of any discomfort and complain that 'the bed is hard' – however soft it may be.

151

Arsenicum Alb. (White Arsenic Oxide)

After *Aconitum*, this is one of the most acute remedies in the repertory – meaning that it is indicated for sudden acute conditions of recent onset. The make-up tends to be the thin restless type, rather fussy and over fastidious to detail. Major symptoms giving the clue to the remedy are overwhelming weakness, collapse and chill. They crave heat and warmth of any kind – either from the fire or hot drinks. In this, the remedy resembles *Rhus tox* which also has much of the restlessness, *Arsenicum* is also deeply agitated in body and mind, often depressed and anxious.

Heat comes into another aspect of the remedy in that burning pains are characteristically coupled with extreme chillness, to the extent of wearing several layers of vests or long-johns on the warmest day. The body heat is always at a low level, and causes the chilly prostration and exhaustion. Diarrhoea with rigors and shivers are frequent.

Belladonna (Deadly nightshade)

This is another invaluable remedy for acute conditions. The typical picture is of redness, inflammation and local heat. The area affected may be the skin as in scarlet fever or erysipelas, or a hang-nail infection spreading up the arm in bright-red inflammatory streaks, with pain and heat along the line of infection. Sensitivity is another important feature with intolerance of the least noise or draught. Movement and jarring causes a most intense aggravation of pain. The sore throat is

152

often worse for swallowing, earache is aggravated by the movement and the skin worse for pressure or touch. An examination may be resisted by floods of tears and all symptoms are increased by lying down. The affected area is often immobilised by lying on it to control movement and pain. Typically the pupils are dilated when there is fever.

Carbo Veg (vegetable charcoal)

Carbo Veg is of enormous value in general sluggish conditions. There is a lack of vital protective energy reaction making the individual slow and vulnerable to whatever infection is currently in the area – so that they are forever 'down' with winter colds, 'flu, coughs or bronchitis. Typically he is tired and irritable with no energy. The great problem is often burning indigestion pains with flatulence or poor circulation. Cold, chill and venous difficulties occur so that the ankles swell easily or varicose veins are marked. It is a most useful emergency remedy for weakness, collapse and faintness – especially for the convalescent patient or when there is fatigue after a period of strain from nursing a sick friend or relative over weeks or months without a break.

Chamomilla (Chamomile)

Chamomilla is an invaluable remedy for the over-sensitive person both physically and mentally. There is a combination of low-pain threshold, irritability, and a grumbling, complaining attitude is generally present – from the young child with

153

teething problems to the adult with unbearable back or menopausal pain. In most cases pain is increased by any form of heat, but a cool local compress brings relief. It is a classic treatment for teething or dental discomfort. Typically the child cries as soon as he lies down and will only sleep or rest when carried. It is important to understand *Chamomilla* as an adult remedy as well as one for teething and it is valuable for a variety of conditions of adult discomfort and unbearable or poorly tolerated painful conditions.

Gelsemium (Yellow Jasmine)

This is one of the best remedies for 'flu conditions, particularly where there is weakness, sluggish exhaustion with trembling and shaking of limbs, often due to rigors as the temperature rises. Indicated also for anxiety conditions, especially examination 'nerves', stage-fright or public-speaking. Weakness of certain muscle-groups as in writer's cramp is relieved. After acute illness and surgery, it stimulates a more rapid return to activity. Most symptoms are aggravated by heat in any form.

Weakness is one of the commonest indications for the remedy. Psychologically they are apathetic and lethargic, paralysed by anxiety or fear. The typical headaches cause exhaustion, the eyes are heavy with no strength in them, the throat weak and feels congested or solid as if there was a lump blocking the area. There is an absence of thirst (compare *Pulsatilla*, *Apis*).

154

Hepar Sulph (Calcium Sulphide)

I recommend this remedy for many of the common infective conditions where there is extreme sensitivity to touch or pressure and when the general disposition is one of anger and irritability. It is useful in throat conditions where there is a splinter-like sensation at the back of the throat and the least exposure to cold dry air aggravates. Cough due to cold, or bronchitis shows this same picture of worsening from cold air and irritability, indicating the remedy. Many skin infective conditions are helped, especially where there is itching, ulceration, or a cheesy-like discharge. Constipation is common and adds to the general picture of impatience and intolerance.

The common psychologicals are a combination of irritability and depression. It is extremely valuable for infective conditions of the eyes where it is useful for Iritis, also for external or middle-ear infections, for erysipelas and in throat conditions – as tonsillitis or quinsy. Splinter-like pain in the area affected is an indication to prescribe.

Hypericum (St. John's Wort)

One of the most important of all the first-aid remedies. It is especially indicated in the treatment of all wounds – both externally as a tincture or cream and internally in the 6th potency. The characteristic picture for prescribing is tenderness and soreness with pain where bleeding has occurred in a puncture or more open wound, especially one involving peripheral nerve damage lead-

155

ing to shooting pains radiating up the limbs. Such injuries may follow a crushed finger tip or a blow to the shin where there is a minimum of protective covering. All symptoms are relieved by warmth and aggravated by cold which intensifies the pain, causing spasm and loss of function in the area. Discomfort is generally intensified by movement or examination of the part affected.

Kali Bic. (Potassium Bichromate)

This remedy has an important role to play in problems of congestion of mucous membrane anywhere in the body. It is particularly helpful in acute or chronic nasal and throat problems with the blockage provoking a stringy, mucus or jelly-like discharge. Troublesome problems of leucor-rhoea are also relieved. Typically the discharges have a yellowish discolouration and the general condition is relieved by warmth and fresh air.

Ledum (Marsh tea)

I recommend this remedy for penetrating wounds and injuries where there is not much pain or sensitivity associated – otherwise *Hypericum* is more needed. The wound is usually clean as from a bite or where a pin or nail has pierced the skin, the area freezing cold – like ice and with a characteristic purplish or bluish tinge to the surrounding skin. Paradoxically, although the surrounding area is so cold, the patient is intolerant of any form of heat and craves a cool atmosphere for comfort. The long-term results of old puncture-wounds still causing discomfort and pain are often relieved by *Ledum*, sometimes many years after the original trauma.

A skin remedy par excellence, particularly useful for insect stings – mosquito, horse-fly, bee or wasp when there is a local inflammation, bruising, pus-formation from a boil or whitlow. The emotional state is a combination of rage or irritability. Like *Natrum mur* there is a desire for solitude as all consolation irritates. Hypersensitivity is marked with the least pressure, movement or touch aggravating the condition. Local inflammation is relieved by a cold pack.

Lycopodium (Club moss)

Inert until made up into its homoeopathic potency, *Lycopodium* is of greatest value for the intellectual type of make-up with little tendency to physical exercise or muscular development. The mind is always strong and active, full of ideas and plans but the body is like an anchor and a barrier to achievement. A remedy for all right-sided problems with typical early afternoon or evening aggravation of all symptoms. There are many chest, throat, kidney and digestive problems most of them beginning on the right side and only later causing trouble on the left. The skin is nearly always dry and sweating is rare. Nervousness and lack of confidence is common and it rivals *Gelsemium* for panic problems, especially where there is an audience or something new and unfamiliar on the horizon. But there are not usually any great problems on the day itself and they nearly always give a good account of themselves – because they also need to be achievers.

Magnesia Phosphorica (Phosphate of magnesium)

Mag. phos. is invaluable for all conditions where pain is associated with spasm and colic. The underlying condition may be intestinal or gall-bladder colic which typically doubles-up the patient. It is improved by local heat but aggravated by cold or draughts. Firm pressure also gives relief and this combined with a hot water bottle may be the only way to obtain relief until *Mag. phos.* is given.

Natrum Muriaticum (Sodium chloride)

This is one of the deepest acting of all homoeopathic remedies, especially in the mental sphere where for many conditions it is unrivalled. It is a remedy for the isolated and solitary, always worse for company because contact with others causes an aggravation of their problems – whether the watery diarrhoea, migraine headaches, or the depression. Easily tearful, walking in a wind, coughing or laughter nearly always brings a flow of tears. Excessive salt is responsible for the common problem of water-retention, clearly seen by the bloated face, fluid under the eyes and often swelling of ankles due to circulatory weakness. Many of their painful complaints are the direct result of the tendency to retain fluid and a disturbed internal salt balance. Most conditions are better for firm local pressure – as the low back pain or ache. In general

158

the sea has either a tonic effect and brings an improvement or alternatively leads to further aggravation.

Nux Vom. (Poison nut)

Another of the greatest remedies in the homoeopathic repertory. It is indicated for the over-worked, over-fed executive, worn-out by work and the pressures of travel, worry and generally 'burning the candle' at both ends. Because of the typical *Nux* temperament, they can do nothing in reasonable moderation, acting impatiently and zealously – too involved emotionally to reach reasonable and rational conclusion and rarely able to see when they are over-tired. Because of their temperament, they are unable to delegate responsibilities either, being typically perfectionistic and demanding of themselves as well as of others around them. They make difficult or 'impossible' unpopular bosses because they can give nobody any initiative without constantly checking and interfering. Their difficulties are nearly always the result of underlying tension and spasm, so that often they have problems of chronic back pain, indigestion or constipation with spasm, worse for noise, pressure and any demand. They are their own worst enemy in most areas.

Phosphorus

The range of action of this remedy is quite extraordinary. It is especially useful for intermittent complaints where there are brief flashes of pain, cough or discomfort. There is nearly always great restlessness and nervousness, the person typically pale, thin, sensitive, and fearful, needing constant reassurance. The remedy acts on all bright red haemorrhagic conditions of any type from piles to a sudden nose-bleed or for deeper disturbances like ulcerative colitis when the overall picture and temperament fits. Usually there is a craving for ice-cold drinks and thirst is intense. *Phosphorus* acts deeply on nearly all the tissues but is pre-eminent in chest problems from asthma to whooping cough and bronchitis. Whenever there are severe chronic problems with breakdown of tissue, even bone – as with a degenerative condition of a bed-ridden elderly person, *Phosphorus* is often the answer. It acts vigorously on the liver and is a remedy to learn and to know in all its actions. The results can be outstanding in conditions that will respond to no other treatment.

Sepia (Ink of the cuttle fish)

A remedy for fatigue and depression especially where there is irritation and a need to get away from others – however close. The patient is typically angry, aggressive, worn-out and dragged-down by their chronic pains and suffering. There is an aching low-back, constipation, period problems with flooding, or exhausting low pelvic pains. All symptoms are better for rest, warmth and frequently for dancing. There is nothing they enjoy more than a brisk walk or exercise – once they can be persuaded to participate. Without *Sepia*, improvement is inevitably short-lasting and rest leads quickly to yet more tiredness and irritability.

This is an important remedy of deep action. It is particularly useful for the treatment of menstrual and uterine disorders including prolapse. Sadness, depression, loss of interest and weakness are the major features. Emotional disturbances are common but it is difficult to cry although this would give relief. There is a sense of being pulled down by life in general. The skin is yellow, with a blotchy discolouration or a saddle-shaped brown marking across the root of the nose.

Sulphur

Sulphur is one of the major remedies for chronic problems which have resisted all other treatment – even homoeopathic ones. Chronic infection is common, especially of the skin with eruptions and a discharge of pus, invariably offensive and dirty-looking. The patient is exhausted, untidy, intolerant of heat or cold and typically made worse by bathing and water. Usually in a muddle, they are full of bright ideas which never materialise or just unrealistic ones. Heat is a major problem and he always feels too hot, or sweats profusely. Indigestion is common with burning-type pains. Many chronic infections are helped by *Sulphur* especially when the skin is also involved. Quickly exhausted and constantly hungry, food is often the only thing that gives comfort or relief. Fats are particularly liked, in spite of the offensive indigestion and diarrhoea that inevitably follows.

161

Thuja (Tree of Life)

Thuja is the remedy to use for the ill-effects of vaccination, even if these occurred many years previously. It is also the recommended treatment for chronic warts of any part of the body – but especially the anal or genital areas. The skin has a most profuse, offensive sweat so that the feet tend to feel 'damp' inside both socks and shoes. Another problem area that *Thuja* helps is a chronic bladder problem – like cystitis, urethral discharges, irritation and recurrent frequency. The added presence of cauliflower-like chronic warts almost certainly confirms the prescription.

Thuja is indicated for deep-seated recurrent problems, the patient usually of swarthy appearance with dark hair and an oily skin. Typical symptoms are localised pains which feel as if a nail has been driven through the area. Also helpful for recurrent infections, neuralgia, nasal catarrh, toothache, throat ulceration and rheumatism.

CHAPTER SIXTEEN

Useful addresses and places of contact

Ainsworth's Homoeopathic Pharmacy,
38, New Cavendish Street, London W1M 7LH.
01 935 5330

Bristol Homoeopathic Hospital
Cotham, Bristol 6.
Bristol 312231

The British Homoeopathic Association
27a, Devonshire Street, London W1N 6BY.
01 935 2163

Baillieston Clinic (Glasgow)
Buchanan Street, Baillieston, Glasgow G69 6DY

Department of Homoeopathic Medicine
The Mossley Hill Hospital, Park Avenue,
Liverpool, L18
051 724 2335

Faculty of Homoeopathy
The Royal London Homoeopathic Hospital
Great Ormond Street, London WC1N 3HR
01 837 8833 Ectn. 85

Freeman's Homoeopathic Pharmacy
7, Eaglesham Road, Clarkston, Glasgow.
041 644 1165

Galen's Homoeopathic Pharmacy
1, South Terrace, South Street, Dorchester,
Dorset.
Dorchester 63996

Glasgow Homoeopathic Hospital
1000 Great Western Road, Glasgow G12 0NR
041 339 0382

Glasgow Out-Patients Clinic
5 Lynedock Crescent, Glasgow G3 6EQ
041 332 4490

Gould's Homoeopathic Pharmacy
14, Crowndale Road, London NW1 1TT.
01 388 4752

The Hahnemann Society
Avenue Lodge, Bounds Green Road, London
N22 4EU
01 889 1595

The Homoeopathic Development Foundation
19A, Cavendish Square, London W1M 9AD
01 629 3204

The Homoeopathic Trust
Hahnemann House, 2 Powis Place, Great Ormond
Street, London WC1N 3HT
01 837 9469

Liverpool Homoeopathic Clinic
Mossley Hill Hospital.
051 724 2335

Manchester Homoeopathic Clinic
Brunswick Street, Ardwick, Manchester.
061 273 2446

Nelson's Homoeopathic Pharmacy
73 Duke Street, Grosvenor Square, London W1M
6BY.

Nelson's Manufacturing Laboratories
5 Endeavour Way, London SW19 9UH
01 946 8527

Royal London Homoeopathic Hospital
Great Ormond Street, London WC1N 3HR
01 837 7821

Tunbridge Wells Homoeopathic Hospital
Church Road, Tunbridge Wells.
0982 42977

Weleda (U.K.) Ltd.
Heanor Road, Ilkeston, Derbyshire DE7 8DR.
0602 303151.

Recommended reading

50 Reasons for being a Homoeopath
J. Compton Burnett

Lectures on Homoeopathic Philosophy
J. T. Kent

Materia Medica
J. T. Kent

Leaders in Homoeopathic Therapeutics
E. B. Nash

Homoeopathic Drug Pictures
M. C. Tyler

First-Aid Homoeopathy
D. M. Gibson

The Patient, Not the Cure
M. G. Blackie

Index

Aconitum, 23, 120, 150
Action of homoeopathy, 75, 78
Acute problems, 59
Addresses, useful, 163
Advantages of homoeopathy, 94
Aesculus hipp., 25
Aethusa, 66
Aggravation, homoeopathic, 33
Agnus cast., 1
Ailanthus, 5
Allergy, 42, 65
Allium cepa, 148
Alumina, 66, 139
Ambra grisea, 2
Ammonium carb., 5
Antimonium crud., 71
Antimonium tart., 140
Apis, 3, 12
Argenticum nitricum, 12
Arndt–Schultz law, 89
Arnica, 24, 119, 151
Arsenicum alb, 16, 23, 152
Attitudes and health, 28
Aurum met, 3, 23

Autumn remedies, 25
Avena sat, 1, 142

Balance and health, 23
Balancing role of hom., 75
Baptisia, 140
Baryta carb., 30
Basic materials of hom., 1
Basic remedies, 150
Belladonna, 4, 7, 8, 12, 30, 52
Bellis perennis, 24, 135, 137
Berberis, 3
Black eye, 134
Blatta, 1
Boils, 134
Bothrops, 2
Breathlessness, 149
Bruises, 137
Bryonia I, 37

Cactus grand, 3
Calcarea, 25, 47
Calendula, 1, 121, 133
Cancer, 107
Cantharis 3, 32

Carbo veg., 39
Casualty conditions, 67
Causation of disease, 36
Caulophyllum, 71
Causticum, 23
Cedron maj., 1, 3
Cenchis contortox, 2
Centreing function of hom., 84
Chamomilla, 153
Childbirth, 71
Childhood complaints, 129
China, 40
Chronic illness, 73, 100, 129, 130
Circulation remedies, 3
Civilisation diseases, 106
Cocculus, 144
Coffea, 146
Colds, 148
Colic, 144
Convallaria maj., 1, 3
Consultation, hom., 100
Contents, v
Controversy, hom., 6
Corallium, 2
Crocus sat, 24
Crotalis horridus, 2
Cuprum met., 115
Curative function of hom., 83
Cuts and wounds, 133
Cyclamen, 25

Deficiency conditions, 71
Definitions, 1
Diet and disease, 54
Diet and homoeopathy, 19, 104
Digitalis, 1, 3, 23
Dilution, 89
Dilution, centisimal, 91

Dilution, decimal, 91
Dilution, Hahnemannian, 116
Dilution, Korsakov, 117
Diphtherinum, 2, 30
Disease, 21
Dulcamara, 2, 11, 23
Dynamic function of hom., 86

Ear, acute problems, 145
Elderly, problems of, 129
Energy reserves, 23
Environmental factors in disease, 56
Epidemic factors in disease, 44
Excretory remedies, 3
Exhaustion, 40, 69

Fainting, 138
Falls and sprains, 135
Ferrum met, 71, 115
First-aid, 66, 110, 133
Fluoric ac., 146
Folic ac., 71
Folliculinum, 71
Foreign bodies, 134
Formica rufa, 1, 71
Fucus vesiculosus, 2

Gelsemium, 24, 113, 154
Ginseng, 138
Graphites, 144

Hahnemann, 14
Hamamelis, 25
Hang-over, 142
Headache, 143
Health of family and hom., 109
Helleborus, 25, 101
Hepar sulph, 25, 101

168

Hiccough, 138
Hippocrates, 15
Holistic approach, 127
House dust, 66
Hydrastis, 155
Hyoscyamus, 64
Hypericum, 46, 133, 155

Iatrogenic factors in disease, 48
Ignatia, 12, 101
Illness, 25, 26, 29
Imbalance and disease, 29
Indications for hom., 59, 106
Indigestion, 140
Infection, 70
Influenzinum, 2, 44
Inherited factors in disease, 37
Insect remedies, 1
Introduction, ix
Ipecacuanha, 31
Ischador, 108

Kali bich., 156
Kreosotum, 139

Lachesis, 2, 5, 12
Laterality of remedies, 125
Latrodectus mactans, 1
Ledum, 134
Lilium tig., 1
Limitations of hom., 103
Lobelia, 140
Lumbago, 147
Lycopodium, 3, 23, 64, 157

Magnesia carb., 140
Magnesia phos., 158
Mechanical factors in disease, 45

Medusa, 2
Medorrhinum, 2, 11, 23
Mental attitudes and disease, 11
Mental illness, 63
Mercurius, 19, 48
Miasms,
Mobility remedies, 2
Morbillinum, 2, 72
Mother substance, 3
Murex, 2
Muriaticum ac., 5
Mygale lasiodora, 1

Naja trip, 2, 23
Natrum mur., 3, 12, 158
Natrum sulph, 3, 23
Nitric ac., 145
Nose bleeding, 137
Nosodes, 2
Nux moschata, 40
Nux vomica, 122, 159

Opium, 23
Organ remedies, 2
Origins, of hom., 3, 14
Overall approach of hom., 8

Paracelsus, 15, 16
Parotidinum, 72
Parasitic factors in disease, 47
Pertussin, 2
Petroleum, 144
Phosphoric ac., 41
Phosphorus, 3, 23, 159
Plant remedies, 1
Plantago, 140
Platina, 125
Plumbum met, 23, 41, 48

169

Podophyllum, 134
Poisoning factors in disease, 48
Pregnancy, 71
Preparation of hom. remedies, 115
Preservative function of hom., 79, 109
Preventative action of hom., 98, 113
Prevention of disease, 72
Provings, 5, 6
Psora, 18
Psorinum, 140
Psychological illness, 24, 59
Psychological factors in illness, 42
Psychological aspects of the remedy, 125
Puerperium, 72
Pulex irritans, 1
Pulsatilla, 1, 3, 11, 12, 13, 23
Pyrogen, 66

Ranunculus bulb, 24
Ratanhia, 138
Recommended reading, 166
Repertory, 7
Resonance, 95
Respiratory remedies, 2
Rhododendron, 2, 11, 23
Rhus tox, 2, 4, 11, 12, 23, 122
Rubellinum, 2
Ruta grav, 2

Santonin, 47
Sea remedies, 2
Sea-sickness, 144
Selenium 66
Sepia, 2, 160

Side-effects of hom., 97
Snake remedies, 2
Social factors in disease, 50
Spigelia, 3, 23
Spongia tost, 23
Spring remedies, 24
Staphisagria, 68, 125
Storage of remedies, 117
Stramonium, 4, 60, 64
Strengthening action of hom., 77
Stress factors and disease, 55, 130
Succussion, 116
Sulphur, 12, 13, 161
Sulphuric ac, 138
Summer remedies, 25
Supportive function of hom., 78
Sycosis, 19
Sycotico, 85
Symphytum, 134
Symptoms, 30, 31, 35
Symptoms, negative, 34

Tabacum, 61
Taking the remedies, 104
Tarentula hisp., 1
Teething problems, 2, 128
Tellurium, 47
Temperature (raised), 142
Tensions, unresolved, 29
Teucrium, 47
Theridon, 1
Throat, acute problems, 145
Thuja, 5, 19, 23, 162
Timothy grass, 66
Toothache, 140
Trachinus, 2
Tuberculinum, 2, 38

170

Unlocking function, of hom., 80
Urticaria, 12, 32

Varicellinum, 2, 72
Vital resources, 95
Vomiting, 139

Winter remedies, 25

X-ray, 33

Zincum met., 115
Zincum met., 115

171